CLINICAL CONTRACEPTION

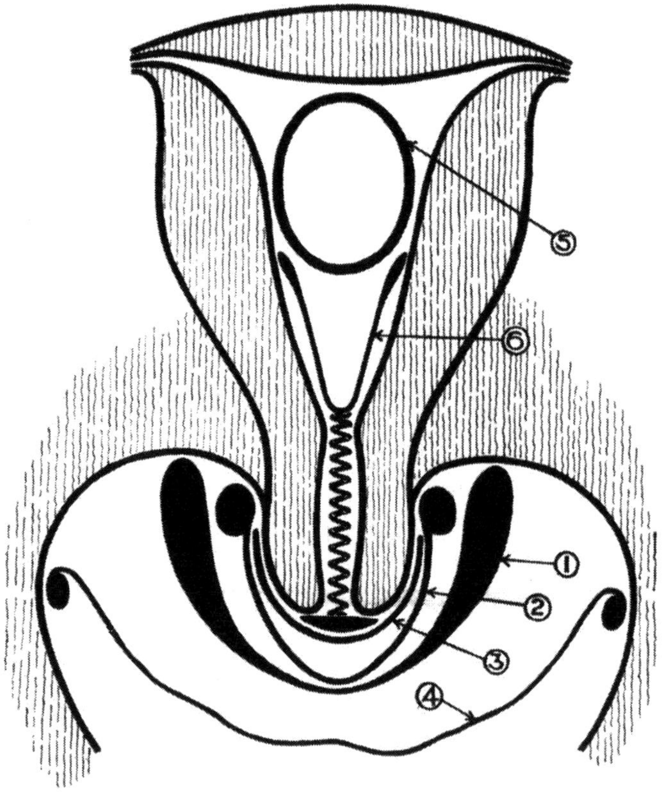

Diagram to Illustrate Types of Mechanical Contraceptives

(*Not drawn to scale*)

1. Dumas pessary. 2. Racial pessary. 3. Portio cap. 4. Dutch or Mensinga pessary. 5. Intra-uterine ring. 6. Wish-bone stem pessary.

Frontispiece.

CLINICAL CONTRACEPTION

By

GLADYS M. COX, M.B., B.S.

Medical Officer to the Society for the Provision of Birth Control Clinics

Member of the Birth Control Investigation Committee

Medical Officer (Part-time) for Maternity and Child Welfare, Greenwich.

INTRODUCTION BY

LORD HORDER OF ASHFORD, K.C.V.O., M.D., F.R.C.P.

SECOND EDITION

LONDON

WILLIAM HEINEMANN

(MEDICAL BOOKS) LIMITED

1937

Printed in Great Britain by
The Whitefriars Press Ltd., London and Tonbridge

INTRODUCTION

THE literature of the subject of Birth Control grows rapidly. A great deal of it deals with the more controversial aspects of the matter; very little of it is essentially practical. But a large section of the public has accepted the principle and considers it already overdue that we move on from the rather casual, if not haphazard, practices to which we have been so long accustomed to something more worthy of the science and art which are supposed to characterise other branches of modern medicine. This rapidly growing clientele expects, and has a right to expect, that the doctor shall be able to give appropriate advice when consulted, and, more than this, that he or she shall demonstrate familiarity with the methods employed and be able to practise them.

This being so, a book which waives argument and at once "gets down to" the practice of Contraception, which is, in other words—as its title describes—"clinical" in its purpose and in its matter, is welcome.

The author's experience is large; her qualification for the task is therefore undoubted. Dr. Cox tells me that she was in some doubt whether to make her instructions limited, concise and dogmatic, or to give a full choice of alternatives to the practitioner, at the same time stating the pros and cons of the various contraceptive methods available. Seeing that the book is written for doctors and to serve as a guide to the complete application of the principle in general practice, I think the decision to adopt the latter course is amply justified. Birth Control, in its clinical significance, is a new branch of medicine; experience of it is growing daily; there is as yet no perfect method; the time has therefore not arrived when dogmatism is legitimate. In view of all this the medical reader should be presented with all the facts and not merely with a few of them. "Type" cases are, however, given in full in these pages, and the method of election in each one of these is stated with lucidity and precision according to the author's experience and judgment.

I feel sure that Dr. Cox's book will supply the information which many practitioners have needed, and I wish it the success which I am confident it deserves.

HORDER.

FOREWORD TO THE FIRST EDITION

I have written this book at the suggestion of the National Birth Control Association. To all who have helped me in various ways, I render my deepest thanks.

I feel it wise to state that I have no commercial or other interests in any of the proprietary contraceptives mentioned in this book.

G. M. COX.

London, 1933.

FOREWORD TO THE SECOND EDITION

On the appearance of this revised edition, I should like to emphasise my conviction that the use of a *combination* of a chemical and a mechanical contraceptive, selected for the individual patient, gives the greatest possible security against conception. The claims made by the manufacturers and distributors of the absolute reliability of certain chemical contraceptives cannot be substantiated clinically.

G. M. COX.

London, 1937.

CONTENTS

CLINICAL CONTRACEPTION

CHAPTER I

INTRODUCTORY

Definition.—The term contraception is here used to cover any modification of normal coitus which has for its object the prevention of pregnancy, either by preventing the fertilisation of the ovum, or by preventing the nidation of a fertilised ovum or by temporarily inhibiting ovulation. Efforts to dislodge an embedded ovum are attempts to procure abortion, and should not be confused with contraceptive methods.

Historical.—The rate of increase of population has, apparently, been checked at all times and in every part of the world, either for eugenic or for economic reasons.

Methods of birth control have included vivisection and abortion, as well as a host of less objectionable and—be it said—less reliable methods. To these methods of birth control proper must be added infanticide, which, at some periods and in some parts of the world, has been practised extensively.

Here it is sufficient to emphasise that birth control is not a new idea; what is new is that the empiricism of the past is now being replaced by methods founded upon scientific research. The methods which are in actual use at the present, however, do not involve any great departure in principle from the less barbarous among the methods of the past; but there is justification for hoping that modern research will yield methods of contraception, perhaps involving new principles, which will be a great advance in reliability and in freedom from æsthetic objections.

Characteristics of the Perfect Contraceptive.—1. It should be harmless, both to the couple using it and to any children who may be born subsequently.

2. It should be æsthetically unobjectionable, and require no genital manipulations for the use of appliances or chemicals.

3. It should not interfere with the spontaneity of coitus.

4. It should be well within the means of those who need to use it.

5. It should be absolutely reliable.

6. It should be simple to use—preferably " foolproof."

7. It should be easy to preserve, and not adversely affected by climatic conditions.

Such a contraceptive has not yet been discovered.

Possible alternatives to the present unæsthetic mechanical and chemical methods of contraception may result from a more complete knowledge of the physiology of reproduction. The hormonic control of reproduction, immunisation by the formation of spermatoxins, and the production of a temporary sterility by diet and by physical agents—application of X-rays to the ovaries or testes, or of heat to the testes—are examples of theoretical biological methods upon which research is now being undertaken.

Disadvantages of Present Methods.—No known method of contraception is absolutely reliable, although a high degree of success can be claimed for certain tested methods. Most methods involve trouble and forethought; the " personal factor " is an element in their successful use, and an elaborate or cumbersome technique renders a method likely to be discarded on occasions and prevents it from being generally acceptable. Few contraceptive methods are reasonably cheap for very poor patients, and methods are often discontinued for economic reasons. Æsthetically, methods involving the use of appliances or chemicals are disliked by many women. Although some methods are almost certainly quite harmless, the same cannot be said of many methods in use at present. The best we can say at the moment is that there are contraceptive methods which are almost certainly harmless, which do not interfere with the spontaneity of intercourse, and which are reasonably reliable.

Evaluation of Methods.—The evaluation of contraceptive methods should take into account the primary function of preventing pregnancy, and the secondary characteristic of being generally acceptable to the patient.

Many statistics of the success or failure of contraceptive methods are misleading, because they fail to take into account such relevant factors as natural fertility of husband and wife, frequency of coitus, the relation of coitus to the periods of maximum and minimum fertility, restriction of intercourse to the relatively "safe" period, and pelvic conditions which predispose to sterility.

A contraceptive method is put to the test each time coitus takes place between a normally fertile couple during the period of the viability of the extruded ovum or when the ovum will be extruded within the period of viability of the ejaculated spermatozoa, when conception is possible.

Fertility.—The patient's previous medical history may afford some evidence as to her natural fertility. For instance, if a young couple leading a normal married life have had three or four children at intervals of one and a half to two years, then, provided that their sexual habits remain unchanged, the success of a contraceptive method which they have adopted can only be determined after a period of two years or longer. Those women who have a natural spacing of three or more years require a correspondingly longer trial period of a contraceptive method before success can reasonably be assumed.

Relation of Female Fertility to Age.—The decline of fertility with age, during the child-bearing period, has been investigated statistically by Munzner and Loer (*Zentralbl. f. Gynäk.*, December 8th, 1934). A study of the birth statistics for Prussia revealed that, out of 100 nulliparæ of a given age, the number who will bear children later is

	Per cent.
At age of 15	68
,, ,, 20	66
,, ,, 25	54
,, ,, 30	30
,, ,, 35	11
,, ,, 40	3
,, ,, 45	0·2

Frequency of Coitus.—Enquiries regarding sexual habits

carried out in America [1] show that the frequency of coitus varies from once a day or oftener to less than once a year. Some patients use contraceptives and also restrict intercourse to the " safe period " as an additional safeguard; some combine the use of contraceptives with the practice of coitus interruptus.

Need for Medical Advice.—Birth control, since it affects the mental and physical welfare of married people and of their children, is a matter which must be of deep interest to the medical practitioner; and not until the profession as a whole shoulders its responsibility in this respect will people be properly protected against exploitation and quackery, which frequently lead to definite physical and mental injury. A completely successful marriage is impossible in the absence of a happily adjusted sex life; and in the large majority of cases a satisfactory method of birth control is essential for sex harmony, while in some cases there are medical reasons for avoiding pregnancy.

No one method of contraception is suitable for all married couples, nor for any one couple in all circumstances. The choice of a contraceptive method is governed by—*inter alia*—local pelvic conditions, general health and intelligence and immediate environment.

The actual fitting of a contraceptive appliance and the instruction in its use may be, in certain cases, simple matters which do not require medical skill; *but a medical training is necessary for the choice of a suitable contraceptive method in each particular case, since there may be present pathological pelvic conditions which require treatment, and which may contra-indicate the use of certain methods and influence the choice of the most suitable possible method.*

MEDICAL INDICATIONS FOR THE PREVENTION OF PREGNANCY

Conditions in which pregnancy would endanger the life of the mother or child, or seriously injure the health of the

[1] " A Thousand Marriages," by R. L. Dickinson and Lura Beam (National Committee of Maternal Health). " Factors in the Sex Life of 2,200 Women," by Katharine Bement Davis (Bureau of Social Hygiene).

mother, or risk the inheritance by the child of certain mental or physical diseases are regarded as medical indications for the prevention of pregnancy, either temporarily or permanently. The responsibility of giving a decision as to the wisdom of parenthood in doubtful cases is commonly thrown upon the medical adviser in general practice.

With the advance of knowledge in methods of diagnosis and treatment, the probability is that the number of cases where there are conclusive medical reasons for contraception will be considerably diminished.

The border-line cases which require careful individual consideration cast a grave responsibility upon the physician who is consulted. He must weigh carefully the possible physiological and psychological injury resulting from the denial of parenthood against the risks of pregnancy and childbirth.

Medical contra-indications of pregnancy include the following conditions :—

Organic Heart Disease.—A well-compensated heart may fail under the extra strain of pregnancy and labour ; on the other hand, many diseased hearts retain good compensation throughout pregnancy, labour, and the puerperium. Heart failure in pregnant women is due primarily to mechanical causes, to the combined effects of the increased body weight and blood volume, the upward displacement of the diaphragm, and the raised metabolic rate. A further factor is the presence of active infection. Any cardiac lesion complicated by active rheumatism is a definite contra-indication to pregnancy. The prognosis in any particular case will depend not only upon the reserve power of the heart muscle and the presence or absence of acute infection, but also upon the possibilities of adequate rest and nutrition, and upon the chances of a short and easy labour, with facilities for forceps delivery or Cæsarian section if advisable.

> "All forms of organic heart disease tend to be adversely affected by pregnancy, so that the patient's expectation of life is, to a greater or less extent, diminished."—(Final Report of Departmental Com-

mittee on Maternal Mortality and Morbidity, Ministry of Health, 1932, p. 128.)[1]

Chronic Nephritis.—Pregnancy should be avoided in all cases where there are unmistakable signs of chronic nephritis.

> " The available evidence proves conclusively that the occurrence of pregnancy in a patient who is already the subject of chronic nephritis is a most serious event for the mother, the nephritis being invariably aggravated and the expectation of life shortened."—(Maternal Mortality Report, p. 129.)

Chronic Pyelitis.

Toxæmias of Pregnancy.—A history of pregnancy toxæmia demands careful consideration of the risks which may be incurred in a subsequent pregnancy.

(*a*) *Albuminuria of pregnancy* (pre-eclampsia) is very liable to be repeated in subsequent pregnancies, and recent investigations in this country and in America reveal 50 per cent. of " recurrent toxæmias." Chronic nephritis may be a sequel, and, according to Eden and Holland (" Manual of Midwifery," 1931), " it is much more likely to arise after one or more repeated toxæmic pregnancies than after the first."

(*b*) *Eclampsia.*—It is estimated that 70 per cent. of cases occur in primigravidæ, therefore the liability is much less in subsequent pregnancies. In the British collective investigation (analysed and reported by Eden) the total maternal mortality was 22 per cent.

Eden and Holland (" Manual of Midwifery," 1931), state :

> " It used to be taught that it was rare for eclampsia to recur in subsequent pregnancies, and that one attack actually conferred immunity against the occurrence of another. We now know, as a result of recent observations, carried out in this country, especially by James Young, of Edinburgh, that one attack of eclampsia, far from protecting a patient, leaves her specially liable to the occurrence of toxæmia in subsequent pregnancies. As a result of observing over a number of years a series of

[1] Referred to subsequently as " Maternal Mortality Report."

women who had recovered from one attack of eclampsia, Young and Syne found that 30 per cent. of subsequent pregnancies were toxæmic."

Considering, then, the high rate of maternal mortality, and the remote maternal prognosis following a previous attack, it would appear to be medically unjustifiable to advise subsequent pregnancies.

(*c*) *Toxæmic vomiting* (hyperemesis gravidarum), in contradistinction to neurotic vomiting, is a true toxæmia, marked by albumen in the urine and marked oliguria. A history of toxæmic vomiting in two or more previous pregnancies is a definite contra-indication to further pregnancy; if it has occurred only once previously, the patient may be willing to risk a recurrence; but it should be recognised that prompt termination of the pregnancy may be necessary if symptoms again supervene.

(*d*) *Acute Yellow Atrophy.* In rare cases recovery occurs, but the patient should on no account risk further pregnancies.

Tuberculosis.—According to Rist (E. Rist, *B.M.J.*, August 13th, 1927, p. 247),

> " almost invariably there is an aggravation of symptoms from flaring up and extension of the existing lesions and the appearance of fresh ones."

Pregnancy should be avoided during the active stage of the disease, and for a further period of two years during which the patient has been clinically well, with temperature normal and sputum free from tubercle.

Diabetes.—The Maternal Mortality Report includes diabetes in the list of medical indications for the avoidance of pregnancy.

At the same time the following observations are recorded :—

> " Before the proper dietetic management of diabetes was understood, the effect of pregnancy on the disease was almost always disastrous. Since the introduction of insulin the outlook for mother and child has been transformed."

The Report quotes the following conclusions of Arnold Walker (*Proc. Soc. Med.*, Vol. XXI., Part I., 1927–1928, p. 378) :—

> " (1) that insulin has entirely altered the outlook on diabetes in pregnancy.
> (2) there now seems to be no reason to terminate pregnancy, and no reason why a diabetic should not give birth to a living child.
> (3) there is no special incidence of puerperal infection ; and
> (4) neither does pregnancy seem to have any ill-effect on the diabetic condition.
>
> There is as much need as in pre-insulin days for general care, especially rest, freedom from worry, avoidance of chills, and exposure to infection. From the beginning of pregnancy the patient should be under the care of a physician who will co-operate with the obstetrician."

It would appear from this that pregnancy is not necessarily contra-indicated for those diabetics who can be assured of regular insulin treatment throughout pregnancy, and of proper pre-natal care. However, the possibility of inheritance of the disease, or its transmission, by the child, is a factor to be considered.

Epilepsy.—Although genuine epilepsy is regarded by most authorities as a " functional neurosis," the risk of a transmission of a predisposition may justifiably be regarded as a contra-indication to reproduction. Direct inheritance of epilepsy is not rare, and insanity and neuroses are commonly associated with epilepsy in the direct or collateral family history.

The influence of pregnancy on epileptics or on those with a hereditary predisposition to epilepsy is summarised in the following extract :—

> " Pregnancy may occasionally be the starting point of epilepsy, especially in those who have a family predisposition to it. In those in whom the disease is already established the effect of pregnancy is very variable. Sometimes there seems to be no influence whatever, but

> in a large proportion the fits are increased in frequency and severity. . . . Pregnancy, too, may cause relapse of an epilepsy which has been for some years apparently cured."—(Maternal Mortality Report, p. 130.)

Primary Amentia.—Mental deficiency due to impaired germ cells is a conclusive reason for avoiding reproduction, on account of the hereditary nature of the disease.

Secondary Amentia.—It should be borne in mind that, even where there is reasonable doubt of the hereditary character of the mental disease, an afflicted parent is not likely to provide a suitable environment for the normal development of a child. Cases of secondary amentia need careful individual consideration.

Reproductive Insanity.—Reproductive insanity (insanity arising in connection with pregnancy, delivery or lactation) is not of itself a contra-indication to further pregnancy, *provided that the attack has been mild (acute in onset and of short duration), and provided that there is a favourable environment for the subsequent pregnancy.*

> " Of all forms of insanity, those associated with reproduction are the most prone to recover completely, especially if the disorder has been acute in its onset and has set in shortly after delivery, but Jones (Robert Jones, *Journ. Obst. and Gyn., Brit. Emp.*, 1903, 3, p. 109) states that he has known many such cases end in chronic dementia ; and Whitridge Williams (J. Whitridge Williams, ' Obstetrics,' 6th Edition, Appleton, p. 1120) says that 20 to 40 per cent. of those following infections fail to regain their normal equilibrium. If the onset has been gradual and the form of the insanity is melancholia, the condition is extremely likely to become chronic. According to Saunders (Saunders, *Amer. Journ. Psychiat.*, 1929, 8, p. 669), only about half these cases recover permanently."—(Maternal Mortality Report, p. 126.)

Hyper-thyroidism.—The marked increase of basal metabolism, great acceleration of the pulse and exaggerated excitability of the heart, and other characteristic symptoms, are definite contra-indications to pregnancy.

Hæmophylia.—This is transmitted usually through the female to the male offspring only; so that, although the woman is unlikely to suffer from dangerous post-puerperal hæmorrhage, she should avoid pregnancy on eugenic grounds.

Pelvic Contraction.—Pelvic contraction is a contra-indication if it be of such a degree as to prevent the birth of a living child or to expose the mother to serious injury at the birth.

The patient may be willing to undergo Cæsarian section as an alternative to adopting some method of birth control. There is a difference of opinion among gynæcologists as to the number of Cæsarian operations which can be undertaken with wisdom, but there can be no doubt of the wisdom of allowing a reasonable interval between pregnancies.

Pernicious Anæmia.

Tubal Pregnancy.—The risk of recurrence of tubal pregnancy is said to be about 5 per cent., a risk which the patient may regard as one which may justifiably be taken, particularly if she can be under medical supervision from the first indication of pregnancy.

Venereal Disease (syphilis and gonorrhœa).

Incomplete Recovery from the Effects of a Previous Pregnancy and Labour.—Two years is probably a reasonable minimum interval between births, but the actual optimum interval will depend upon the health of the mother and child, and the economic conditions and general environment of the family. Hegar has stipulated an interval of at least 30 months between pregnancies.

CLASSIFICATION OF METHODS OF CONTRACEPTION

Some methods here included are still in the theoretical stage; and, although experiments are being conducted on animals, these methods cannot yet, and possibly may never, be applied to humans.

Other methods are definitely harmful or completely unreliable, and should not be used.

The remainder, selected for individual cases, and used

correctly in suitable combinations, are moderately reliable and probably harmless.

METHODS OF CONTRACEPTION

I. Biological.—(*a*) *Serological:* the injection of semen to produce temporary sterility through the formation of spermatoxins.

(*b*) Hormonic control of reproductive activity.

(*c*) Temporary arrest of ovulation or spermatogenesis by irradiation of ovaries or testes; or by heat to the testicle.

(*d*) Dietetic control of reproduction.

II. Physiological.

(*a*) Coitus interruptus (withdrawal).

(*b*) Coitus reservatus.

(*c*) Coitus saxonus.

(*d*) Special coital positions to avoid contact of ejaculate and upper vagina.

(*e*) "Safe period"—a phase of complete sterility in the menstrual cycle.

(*f*) Lactation.

III. Chemical (secondary mechanical action).

(*a*) Ointments, creams, jellies.

(*b*) Suppositories.

(*c*) Effervescing tablets and jellies.

(*d*) Douche with spermicidal solution.

(*e*) Lathering.

IV. Mechanical.

(*a*) Condom.

(*b*) Occlusive pessaries—vaginal diaphragms, vault pessaries, cervical caps.

(*c*) Sponges and tampons.

(*d*) Douche—depending upon mechanical action of irrigation.

(*e*) Intra-uterine pessaries—stem pessaries, stars and rings (intra-uterine appliances may in some cases act as abortifacients and not as contraceptives).

Combinations of methods in common use are:—

1. Condom with spermicide (jelly or suppository or foam tablet).

2. Occlusive pessary with spermicidal lubricant and suppository jelly or tablet.
3. Occlusive pessary with spermicidal lubricant and douching.

The *selection* of the combination of methods will be influenced by such factors as :—

1. Local pelvic condition.
2. Frequency of coitus.
3. Degree of protection desired, depending on medical indications for contraception, pelvic condition, previous history of fertility, etc.
4. Æsthetic considerations.
5. Practicability—domestic and economic limitations, intelligence of patient, travel, and climate.

CHAPTER II

PHYSIOLOGY OF REPRODUCTION IN RELATION TO THE PROBLEM OF CONTRACEPTION

In order to comprehend the difficulties and complexities of effective contraception, it is well to consider certain aspects of reproduction which have a definite bearing on the control of conception.

Factors which must be taken into account include the following :—

1. The exact occasions of normal ovulation in relation to the menstrual periods and to the periods during which the extruded ovum is capable of being fertilised.

2. Irregular ovulation, due to endocrine activity and possibly stimulated by orgasm or by emotional causes.

3. The behaviour of the uterus during orgasm (muscular contractions, " dipping," " interlocking " of the cervix and glans penis, extrusion of the mucous plug, insuck of semen).

4. The possibility of direct ejaculation of semen into a dilated cervical os in certain cases of uterine displacement (retroversion, acute ante-flexion), and during certain coital positions wherein the axis of the cervical canal is brought into line with that of the phallus.

5. The length of time sperms can retain their fertilising power within the female genital tract.

6. The rate of movement of sperms in favourable conditions, and the minimum time taken for sperms deposited on the cervix in the region of the os to enter the cervical canal.

7. Variation in the *p*H of vaginal secretions and the effects of that variation upon fertility.

8. The alkalinity of cervical secretions and of semen, which is favourable to spermatozoa.

9. The possible absorption of semen by the vaginal mucous membrane and the effects of such absorption.

10. Effect of hormones (lutein, œstrin, pituitrin, etc.) on reproductive activity.

Ovulation.—It is now generally agreed that the time of ovulation in women varies within fairly wide limits in the menstrual cycle, but there are conflicting views regarding these limits.

Evans and Swezy (*Mem. Univ. Calif.*, IX., p. 119, 1931) maintain that "the ova of adult life are being continually produced and just as continually destroyed." Evans points out that, although in certain mammals (rat, guinea-pig and dog) ovulation is known to occur during the period of secretion of œstrum (the alpha hormone), the conditions are different in man and in monkey, in whom "the follicular cycle has no necessary relation to menstruation, and ovulation takes place at any time after the beginning of menstruation." Bolaffio (*Zentralbl. f. Gynäk.*, June 18th, 1932, p. 1510) also concludes that conception is possible at any time in the menstrual cycle. Knaus (*Zentralbl. f. Gynäk.*, March 19th, 1932, p. 721) considers that ovulation is most likely to occur from the fourteenth to the sixteenth day after the onset of menstruation; and Ogino agrees with him that, in a woman with a twenty-eight-day menstrual cycle, ovulation never occurs during the eleven days preceding menstruation. According to Charles ("The Practice of Birth Control," 1932, pp. 98 and 102), recent study points to the conclusion that ovulation is most likely to occur from the seventh to the thirteenth day after the onset of menstruation. Zuckerman (*Brit. Med. Journ.*, Dec. 17th, 1932, p. 1093) stresses the evidence of the œstrous phenomenon of changes in the sexual skin (subsidence of sexual-skin swelling) as a sign of ovulation in the primate menstrual cycle. He remarks :—

> "In the baboon (genus Papio) the sudden decrease of the swelling about the mid-point of the cycle has been shown to synchronise, apparently closely, with ovulation. The decrease in coloration which usually occurs in the rhesus monkey shortly after the middle of the cycle is also clearly correlated with the time of ovulation determined by direct methods. There can be

little doubt that the same relation applies in other species.

There is thus in the sexual-skin phenomenon a ready indication of the time of ovulation, which has yielded abundant evidence to support the conclusion, arrived at from many other lines of investigation, that ovulation both in man and in subhuman catarrhine primates normally occurs about the middle of the cycle."

Hartman (*Iden. Anat. Rec.*, 1932, lii., p. 14) supplies evidence from the controlled matings of rhesus monkeys. In fifty-eight pregnancies conception occurred between the ninth and the eighteenth day of the menstrual cycle.

Direct observation of the ovaries, recorded by many workers, supports the view that ovulation is generally confined to a small number of days in the middle of the menstrual cycle. There is also reason to think that irregular ovulation may occur at any time in the menstrual cycle as a result of the stimulus of orgasm or from other causes.

The probability is that ovulation occurs normally at a definite stage in the middle of the menstrual cycle, and is followed by a period of luteal activity; but that irregular ovulation may also occur.

The temporary suspension of ovulation occurs during pregnancy, and usually during lactation also. The appearance of menstruation during lactation is regarded as evidence that ovulation has recommenced, but clinical records of conception during lactation show that ovulation may, and frequently does, precede the resumption of menstruation.

Duration of Life of the Extruded Ovum.—A number of medical writers consider that the human ovum remains alive and capable of being fertilised in the genital tract for periods as long as fifteen days after ovulation. We have no direct evidence on this point, but by analogy with the mammalian species whose ova are known to survive for periods varying from two to ten hours, the duration of life of the unfertilised human ovum is almost certainly very much less than this estimate and probably not more than twenty-four hours.

Coitus.—During coitus, the erect penis ejaculates seminal fluid into the vagina. The pre-ejaculatory mucoid secretion from the urethral glands acts as a lubricant, and facilitates the intromission ; in the female a similar mucoid secretion from the vulvo-vaginal vestibulary glands (Skene's and Bartholin's) and in the upper vagina from the cervical glands, is produced in response to adequate sexual stimulation. This secretion is diminished or absent in women who are actually or apparently frigid, or whose vaginal and cervical mucous membranes have been injured by the excessive use of astringent douches or other chemicals ; and *in such cases of diminished secretion one would not recommend the use of a chemical spermicide, such as a foam tablet, which depends upon a normal amount of vaginal moisture for its efficacy.*

Penetration is followed by coital movements, accompanied by increasing excitement which, after a period—which may vary between extremes of about one minute or less in cases of premature ejaculation and twenty minutes or more in prolonged intromission, about five minutes being the normal —culminates in orgasm, when the semen is ejaculated in a series of jets. After detumescence and the withdrawal of the penis, most of the semen ultimately flows out of the vagina, but even one droplet, caught up in a fold of vaginal mucous membrane, may contain many thousands of motile sperms, each capable of propelling itself along the moist mucous membrane to the cervix and into the uterus, in which process it is assisted by chemical attraction. *Conception is favoured if the ejaculate is deposited on or near the os*—because of the favourable alkalinity of cervical secretions and because of the proximity of the cervical canal, in which sperms are out of reach of vaginal spermicides—and the use of an occlusive pessary aims at preventing this from occurring. The exact site in which the seminal fluid is deposited depends not only upon the degree of penetration, but also upon the relation of the vaginal axis to the direction of movement of the phallus. The longer the semen remains within the vagina—within the limit of the duration of life of the spermatozoa—the greater is the chance of conception. The degree of penetration may be limited voluntarily for contraceptive purposes; it is also limited by the relative length of the phallus. Certain variations from the habitual median attitude of the converse (face to face) position favour contraception by directing the ejaculate away from the upper vagina.[1]

> For contraceptive purposes, Van de Velde advises that in positions where complete penetration is effected, as in the habitual medial attitude of the converse (face to face) position, the phallus should be deflected before ejaculation. Attitudes in which conception is least likely include the second attitude of the converse position (female supination), and the fifth attitude of the converse position (sedentary—face to face).

Orgasm in the female is preceded by a crescendo of sensation, accompanied by hyperæmia of the vulvo-vaginal and uterine tissues and by the production of a lubricating secretion from the vulvo-vaginal and cervical glands. The alkaline cervical mucus preserves and invigorates spermatozoa; and there is evidence that it may protect them from the spermicidal action of certain chemical contraceptives.

Unfortunately, the pre-orgasmal period is normally considerably shorter in the male than in the female. The lack of synchronisation is most marked in those cases of premature ejaculation and of coitus interruptus where the intromission period is not sufficiently prolonged to allow the wife to reach orgasm. It also occurs where the wife's sexual response is markedly subnormal, either through faulty coital technique (insufficient preliminary wooing and stimulation of the erotic zones), or through dyspareunia, ill-health, exhaustion or any other cause.

When a woman is sexually aroused in coitus, but fails to experience orgasm, the normal detumescence of the uterine and surrounding tissues does not occur; sexual desire persists, and leads to post-coital restlessness and psychic distress. There is evidence that such a condition of affairs persisting over a period may lead to pelvic disorders

[1] For full details of coital positions, see Van de Velde's "Fertility and Sterility in Marriage," pp. 304–314, and "Ideal Marriage," Ch. XI.

associated with chronic congestion, to neurasthenic symptoms, and ultimately to frigidity.

Any contraceptive method is unsatisfactory if it tends to lessen the sexual response of the wife, and therefore postpones or inhibits her orgasm, or which otherwise interferes with the normal course of coitus.

Behaviour of the Uterus during Orgasm.—The behaviour of the uterus during orgasm has an important bearing on problems of contraception. At present there is difference of opinion on this point among gynæcologists. According to Van de Velde (" Fertility and Sterility in Marriage," p. 113) :—

> " . . . the orgasmic contractions of the uterus act as a kind of suction pump, and the organ alters its position, so that the outer extremity of the cervix (the so-called exterior os) is dipped into the seminal lake. The Kristeller, or dense mucous plug in the external os, may protrude itself into the seminal fluid and slip back into its normal position, covered with spermatozoa, which are thus introduced into the womb."

Regarding the descent of the uterus during orgasm, Dickinson and Bryant (" Control of Conception," p. 33) remark that :—

> " There is in woman no anatomical machinery to bring about descent except pressure from the abdominal muscles, and this drives the entire contents of the pelvis downwards and not the uterus alone. There are several such observations recorded, but there are more well-accredited case histories of observed orgasm without evidence of descent."

There is some evidence, from direct observation of the cervix during orgasm, which supports the view that rhythmic movements of the cervix do occur in some cases. Munde has noted the external os opening and closing slightly, with ejection of cervical mucus, during orgasm ; and Dickinson records one case of " opening and closing," and has found " softening during examination on rare occasions."

"Talmey and Beck have recorded 'outroll and inroll of the lips of the cervix and outpour and insuck of secretion in repeated and striking rhythm.' A swaying of the cervix in pendulum swings occurred in Talmey's external os, 'just passable for an ordinary uterine sound,' and opening 'to admit the index finger' for three gasps, five times in twelve seconds; while in the Beck instance, the 'firm, hard' normal cervix with 'the os closed so as not to admit the uterine probe without difficulty,' is said to have opened to the extent of fully an inch, made five or six successive gasps, drawing the external os into the cervix powerfully, all in twelve seconds."—("Control of Conception," p. 34.)

Such powerful action of the cervix, with insuck of semen, would naturally favour conception, and any contraceptive method in such cases must include a mechanical barrier to prevent direct insemination during orgasm. Yet many women who never experience orgasm have a high fertility rate—a common history in birth control clinics. It may be that, in many of these cases of diminished or absent sex feeling, the uterus is so placed as to bring the cervical canal into the line of axis of the vagina, so that the semen is sprayed directly upon the region of the os; certainly in some cases the cervix is so relaxed, owing to childbirth injuries or to general lack of tone, that semen may be ejaculated directly into the cervical canal. Even in the absence of orgasm, such a physical condition of the uterus would facilitate conception.

Stopes ("Contraception," p. 234, 3rd Ed.) maintains that there may be definite "interlocking" of the glans penis and the cervix. She differentiates two types of women in which this may occur: (1) "the passive and large os, which is so much stretched that it remains open voluntarily, permitting the easy penetration, sometimes of one finger and sometimes even of two fingers," and (2) "an os normally closed, which is capable of opening under the stress of sexual excitation to permit the interlocking with the glans penis."

Jay reported that a portion of a condom, torn from the penis during coitus, was found within the cervical canal.

> "The following case is interesting, as it seems to throw light on the action of the cervix uteri during coitus. I was called to see a woman who informed me that one hour previously, during coitus, a part of the sheath worn by her husband was torn away, and remained in the vagina, whence she could not remove it. On examination I found the sheath firmly fixed in the cervical canal; some force was required to pull it out. About 2 inches of the sheath was in the canal, I think the tip must have passed through the internal os. I examined the woman the following day; the cervix was quite healthy and the cervical canal would not permit the passage of a fine probe."—(Letter to *Brit. Med. Journ.*, August 10th, 1929.)

The interpretation of this fact has given rise to some controversy; definite "interlocking" may have occurred, followed by a powerful contraction of the cervix, which gripped a loose portion of the condom as the penis was withdrawn; or the teat end of the condom may have been sucked into the cervix during an orgasm similar to that observed by Beck (quoted above).

At the suggestion of the Birth Control Investigation Committee, investigations have been conducted by Drs. H. M. Carleton and H. M. Florey to determine whether substances in the vagina are aspirated or forced into the uterus during coitus.

Experiments were made as follows:—

1. Injection of Pigment under Pressure into the Vagina.—The pigment used was hydrokollag, a fine suspension of graphite. The vaginal aperture was tightly held round the nozzle of a syringe during the injection.

(*a*) *Rabbits.*—The suspension of pigment was injected with sufficient pressure to balloon the vagina. On no occasion was pigment found above the external os.

(*b*) *Rats.*—Pigment was found in the uterus after sudden and forcible injection; but with slow injection, even with the attainment of high pressure, the suspension of pigment did not enter the uterus.

(*c*) *Dogs.*—As in the case of rabbits, it was found impossible to inject the pigment into the uterus from the vagina.

2. Injection of Pigment before and during Coitus.—(*a*) *Rabbits.*—The seminal vesicles of rabbits were injected with

the pigment hydrokollag twenty-four hours before copulation. It is noted that "sexual vigour seemed unimpaired, and the pigment was ejaculated without loss." Although sperms were sometimes found in the uterus, the pigment was in all cases localised in the vagina.

(*b*) *Dogs.*—At the moment of intromission, a charge of pigment suspension was injected into the vagina in the region of the external os through a catheter previously attached in position. No pigment was found above the external os after coitus.

The following conclusions are reported :—

> "1. It is impossible (except under certain conditions in the rat) to force material from the vagina into the uterus.
>
> 2. Not any substances are either aspirated or injected from the vagina into the uterine cavity during coitus in rabbits.
>
> 3. By somewhat indirect methods a similar conclusion is reached for the dog, viz., that material in the vagina does not gain entrance to the uterus during coitus.
>
> 4. It is therefore clear that, though the presence of sperms in the uterus may be noted soon after coitus, such presence can only be ascribed to the intrinsic motility of the male germ cells.
>
> 5. It is admitted that these results are the outcome of experiments on two widely different species whose organs of generation differ somewhat from those of man. It must be conceded, however, that these results should be applied to the human beings until, or unless, quite unequivocal evidence to the contrary is produced."

"Birth Control Studies. 2. On the Ingress of Semen into the Uterus during Coitus." H. M. Carleton and Howard Florey. *Journ. of Obstet. and Gynæc. of the British Empire*, Vol. 38, No. 3.

Walton and other research workers also concluded, from observations on animals whose vaginæ were filled with coloured fluid immediately before coitus, that fluids do not pass from the vagina into the uterus.

The Birth Control Investigation Committee, recognising the variation in reproductive mechanisms in different species, has devised a method, requiring the co-operation of married couples, of investigating the reactions of the cervix in women.[1]

> A radio-opaque substance (an emulsion of barium) is expressed into the upper vagina before coitus. If contraceptive measures are desired, the husband can wear a sheath or the wife can insert a diaphragm pessary below the barium. A post-coital douche is used to remove all traces of the barium from the vagina. The pelvis is later radiographed to detect the presence of any barium in the cervical canal or uterine cavity.

Effect of Orgasm on Fertility.—It is assumed that orgasm in the female facilitates conception. If orgasm is accompanied by insuck of semen into the uterus, or if in favourable conditions interlocking can take place, with ejaculation directly into the uterus, then the assumption is a reasonable one. One would then expect a much lower rate of fertility in cases of frigidity. Dickinson, however, found only a difference of 2 per cent. in fertility between responsive and frigid women among 1,000 cases observed. Such a close approximation may, perhaps, be explained by the high rate of fertility in women who, although of the frigid type, have the large soft cervix with dilated os and the type of uterine displacement which facilitates direct ejaculation either on to the cervix in the region of the os, or even into the cervical canal. Clinically, it is not uncommon to find women who never experience orgasm and yet have a high fertility rate. Nevertheless, there is considerable evidence that, in the average sexual types of women, orgasm facilitates conception.

It is perhaps not surprising that medical records yield only isolated instances of direct observation of the behaviour of the cervix during a patient's orgasm. The writer has made some thousands of pelvic examinations, but in no case did orgasm occur, so that there was no opportunity of

[1] Full instructions will be sent to any applicant, together with a tube of barium emulsion, a sheath and a vaginal douche, free of charge. The Birth Control Investigation Committee will be very grateful to anyone who will co-operate in this experiment. Communications should be addressed to the Honorary Secretary, Birth Control Investigation Committee, 26 Eccleston Street, S.W. 1.

observing the behaviour of the patient's cervix during orgasm.

It is only to be expected that direct observation of the phenomenon is a very rare experience, but this rarity does not lessen the significance of those cases which have been observed and reported.

Vaginal Secretions and their Effect upon Fertility.—In addition to individual variations in the *p*H of vaginal secretions in health and disease, there is reason to think that there are normal variations in the *p*H of vaginal and cervical secretions during the menstrual cycle of the healthy woman. The exact effect of these variations on fertility has not yet been satisfactorily investigated, but the probability that the effectiveness of contraceptive methods may vary in the normal woman at different periods of the menstrual cycle, and may also be affected by pathological vaginal and cervical secretions, should be kept in mind.

Motility, Longevity and Fertilising Power of Spermatozoa.—The normal site of impregnation, when a spermatozoon fuses with the ovum, is within the Fallopian tube. The upward progress of the sperms from the vagina is facilitated by their motility, by the capillary currents in part of the genital tract, by the favourable alkaline reaction of the cervical mucus, and by chemotaxis. The rate of movement of spermatozoa on a slide is about 3 mm. a minute or about ½ inch in four minutes, but it is considered to be considerably less in the vagina, where a rate of 1½ mm. in three minutes has been estimated. *Sperms deposited in the region of the os may in a very short time be within the cervical canal, out of reach of spermicidal douches, suppositories, tablets or jellies used* after *coitus.*

The longevity of human spermatozoa within the vagina is not definitely known. It probably varies according to special conditions and types of secretion. The normal vaginal acidity (*p*H 3·8–4·5) is inimical to their survival; but the *p*H value of vaginal secretions is a variable factor, and is raised by the alkaline cervical mucus secreted during sexual excitement and by admixture with the volume of alkaline semen, which has a *p*H value 8·5–9. Moreover, the semen itself has a definite buffer action. The acidity of the normal vagina is estimated at 0·5 per cent. of lactic acid ; and, according to several observers, sperms can live for hours in a 0·5 per cent. solution of lactic acid. The probable individual variation in the *p*H of the normal vaginal secretions *within the monthly cycle* is another factor to be considered.

Reynolds and McComber (" Practice of Contraception," Sanger and Stone, p. 11) state that the sperms " seldom survive for more than one to one and a half hours in the normal vaginal pool, and when the vaginal acidity is high they become still within a few minutes." According to Van de Velde (" Fertility and Sterility in Marriage," p. 114) sperms are " so rapidly destroyed by the slightly acid vaginal secretions that there are none living within four hours after emission." Belonoshkin states that living sperms may be found in the vagina for twenty-four hours after coitus (*Arch. f. Gynäk.*, November, 1934). Yet there is some evidence that sperms can live for days within the vagina. Cary (*Jour. Amer. Med. Assoc.*, June 27th, 1936) reports that, in the course of his investigation of cervical mucus, he found in four cases normally migrating sperm cells thirty-six, sixty, sixty-four and eighty hours respectively after the last coitus. An examination of cervical fluid of five patients after artificial insemination with the semen of one donor was made by Seymour (*Jour. Amer. Med. Assoc.*, May 16th, 1936). At the end of three hours the spermatozoa were very active in the cervical fluid of three of the patients, sluggish in one, and dead in another ; at the end of forty-five hours, sperms were still active in one case and sluggish in two others. After ninety hours there were sluggish cells in two cases, and after one hundred and ten hours—the fifth day of insemination—the sperms were still alive in one case. Hühner (*Jour. Amer. Med. Assoc.*, November 7th, 1936) states that he found living spermatozoa in the cervix five days after coitus. Taylor's " Principles and Practice of Medical Jurisprudence " (Vol. 2, p. 952) records cases in which spermatozoa lived in the vagina as long as seventeen days ; and even longer periods are reported. We know that conception can occur in virgins when the semen is deposited outside an intact hymen, and we have clinical evidence that a post-coital douche, accompanying the removal of an occlusive pessary eight or more hours after coitus, is an important contributory factor to the success of this combined method of contraception.

However, the extreme estimates of a longevity of several weeks given in the older medical text-books are rendered highly improbable by the recent studies of Hammond, Walton, Moore and Knaus on the longevity of spermatozoa in certain mammals (rabbit, guinea-pig, and horse) in which the period of survival lies between twelve and twenty-four hours.

Knaus (1932) concluded, as a result of his experimental work on rabbits, that the fertilising power of spermatozoa within the female genital tract persisted not longer than four days.

Moreover, Robson points out that the periods of fertilising capacity and of motility of spermatozoa are not concomitant. He writes: ". . . it has been conclusively demonstrated that, at least in the rabbit, spermatozoa lose their power of fertilisation long before motility disappears" ("Recent Advances in Sex and Reproductive Physiology," p. 126). Thus the data deduced from the recovery of motile sperms from the vagina do not necessarily prove the duration of fertilising power.

The conclusion is that methods of contraception should include not only a mechanical barrier (occlusive pessary) over the cervix, but, in addition, a chemical spermicide (suppository, tablet, jelly or douche) to prevent motile spermatozoa from ascending into the uterus after the cervix has been uncovered by the post-coital removal of the occlusive pessary.

The Seminal Fluid.—This is a mucilaginous mixture composed of from two to five million spermatozoa (which have been stored in the epididymis) suspended in an albuminous fluid composed of secretions from the seminal vesicles and the prostate glands. The high *p*H value (8·5) of these alkaline secretions is the optimum for the maintenance of vitality of spermatozoa; and the secretions may have a definite nutritive and stimulating function in relation to spermatozoa. The average volume of the ejaculate is about 4 c.c., but amounts varying from ¾ c.c. to 30 c.c. have been observed. Cowper's gland and the urethral glands supply a pre-ejaculatory lubricating fluid, which has been demonstrated to contain active sperms in some cases. *This latter fact probably accounts largely for the failure of coitus interruptus as a method of contraception.*

Absorption of Semen.—The possibility of the absorption of substances from the seminal fluid by the vaginal mucous membrane, with beneficial effects upon the woman, has a bearing upon the choice of a contraceptive. Stopes (" Contraception," p. 82) expresses the view that " women absorb from the seminal fluid of man some substance, ' hormone,' ' vitamine,' or stimulant which affects their internal economy in such a way as to benefit and nourish their whole systems " ; and Van de Velde (" Fertility and Sterility in Marriage," p. 325) suggests that there may be a physiological " hunger for the male fluid " in the female organism, analogous to the instinctive hunger for salt, lime, and vitamines. On the other hand, Dickinson and Bryant (" Control of Conception," p. 28), referring to this supposition of the beneficial absorption of semen, remark : " We are yet at sea on this matter, so that this consideration carries no weight at present " ; and Charles (" The Practice of Birth Control," p. 51) states : " No experimental evidence derived from physiological enquiry into mammalian reproduction supports this supposition." However, it is known that certain substances (*e.g.*, quinine, sodium salicylate, potassium iodide, perchloride of mercury, etc.) are absorbed by the vaginal mucous membrane. The supposition that beneficial elements from the seminal fluid can also be absorbed is at least possible, and demands due consideration in evaluating contraceptive methods.

Frequency of Intercourse.—The possibility of conception is probably generally restricted to a definite period during the menstrual cycle—a period limited by the longevity of the extruded ovum and of the spermatozoa in the female genital tract—and the frequency of intercourse during this period has a bearing on the interpretation of statistics of the reliability of contraceptive methods.

Frequency of intercourse must also be taken into consideration in the choice of a method in each case, since a particular chemical contraceptive may be quite harmless used once or twice a week, but inadvisable for daily use.

An enquiry in America (" A Thousand Marriages," Dickinson & Beam, Medical Aspects of Human Fertility Series, issued by the National Committee on Maternal Health) revealed that, in respect of 526 couples, the average frequency of coitus was twice a week. Actual figures are given—daily or oftener, 16 per cent.; two or three times a week, 23 per cent.; one or two times a week, 20 per cent.; once a week, 17 per cent.; fortnightly to monthly, 10 per cent.; once in one to six months, 3 per cent.; once a year or less, 11 per cent.

A publication of the American Bureau of Social Hygiene (" Factors in the Sex Life of Twenty-two Hundred Women," by Katharine Bement Davis) gives the following analysis of the replies of 979 women regarding the frequency of coitus. More than once a day, 2 per cent.; once a day, 7·6 per cent.; more than twice a week, 31·3 per cent.; once or twice a week, 40 per cent.; " often " or " frequently," 2·4 per cent.; " seldom " or " infrequently," 3·9 per cent.

A contraceptive method which is put to the test only three or four times a month is likely to give a higher proportion of successes over a period than when it is used daily over the same period.

Safe Period.—The recognition of an *absolute* " safe period," during which it is impossible for coitus to be fertile, depends upon :—

(*a*) A knowledge of the time of ovulation in relation to menstruation; whether spontaneous irregular ovulation may also occur; the length of time the ovum is capable of fertilisation in the genital tract; and

(*b*) A knowledge of the duration of the fertilising power of the sperms deposited in the vagina.

It is impossible to determine, for any particular woman, the exact date of ovulation; moreover, there is the possibility of the bursting of a follicle and the extrusion of an ovum as a result of the stimulus of coitus or from other causes; and the longevity of and duration of the fertilising power of human spermatozoa within the female genital tract is not yet definitely known.

Knaus ("Ueber den Zeitpunkt der Konzeptionsfähigkeit des Weibes im Intermenstruum," *Munch. Mediz. Wochenschr.*, 76, p. 1157 (July), 1929) maintains that, in the case of a woman with a regular twenty-eight day menstrual cycle, conception can occur only from the eleventh to the seventeenth day, and that physiological sterility obtains during the remainder of this period. Ogino (*Zentralbl. f. Gynäk.*, March 19th, 1932, p. 721) agrees with Knaus that in a woman with a twenty-eight day menstrual cycle the eleven days preceding menstruation constitute a period of sterility.

Even if this be true, however, the fact remains that a substantial proportion of women have irregular menstruation, or a cycle greater or less than the normal twenty-eight days.

Bolaffio (*Zentralbl. f. Gynäk.*, June 18th, 1932, p. 1510) disagrees with Ogino and Knaus on this point. He concludes that conception is possible at any time in the menstrual cycle, but that it is most likely to result from coitus within the first twelve days. The so-called "safe period" of Ogino and Knaus he regards as the period of minimum fertility. Evans and Swezy (*Mem. Univ. Calif.*, IX., p. 119, 1931) conclude that ovulation may take place at any time in the menstrual cycle, thus precluding a definite and regular period of physiological sterility.

Clinical evidence, collected by Dickinson and others, supports the view that *there is no absolute safe period.* In a group of 1,342 cases among women with a twenty-eight-day menstrual cycle, in which the date of an isolated coitus resulting in pregnancy was known, conception occurred presumably on all days of the cycle—37 per cent. in the first week, 35 per cent. in the second week, 20 per cent. in the third week, and 8 per cent. in the fourth week. Thus 72 per cent. of the conceptions occurred in the first two weeks, and the fourth week was the relatively unfertile period.

Schumacher (*Monatsschrift f. Geburtshuelfe u. Gynaekologie*, March, 1935) relates three instances of conceptions which had occurred following an isolated coitus on the third, second and first days respectively preceding the expected onset of menstruation.

In further support of the unreliability of the "safe period" of Ogino and Knaus, the writer has eight patients who have regular twenty-eight-day menstrual cycles, and who conceived during the week preceding the onset of menstruation, and one of these conceived as a result of coitus on the first day of menstruation.

The conclusion is, therefore, that *there are periods of maximum and minimum fertility in the menstrual cycle—periods which are probably variable, and which in any case cannot be definitely predicted in any individual case: but there is no absolute safe period. Conception is probably least likely to occur during the ten days immediately preceding the onset of menstruation: and the mid-menstrual period, contrary to former views, represents a period of maximum fertility.* Some patients, whose fecundity is low, may find from experience that restriction of intercourse to the ten days preceding menstruation is adequate for limitation of the family.

Effect of Hormones on Reproductive Activity.—Reproductive activity is controlled by various hormones, and the possibility of producing, without injury to health, a definite revocable sterility by the use of hormones is now being considered.

According to Marshall ("Recent Research on the Sex Hormones and their Cyclical Production," by F. H. A. Marshall, Sc.D., F.R.S., *Brit. Med. Journ.*, August 6th, 1932, p. 232), the œstrous or sexual cycle in man is probably a poly-œstrum or succession of menstrual cycles; and there may or may not also be an anœstrum (resting phase).

The succession of events has been worked out recently on monkeys and baboons (by Corner and Allen, by Hartman, and by Parkes and Zukermann).

1. A well-marked *growth period* preceding menstruation.
2. A *period of destruction,* manifested in the menstrual discharge.

3. A *follicular stage*, followed by ovulation about the fourteenth day after the onset of menstruation.

4. A *luteal phase*—the formation of corpus luteum, commencing an "abbreviated pseudo-pregnancy" (Marshall) which persists up to the commencement of the next menstrual period.

The corpus luteum is not formed if, as may happen, ovulation does not occur during the cycle.

Ovarian Hormones

(*a*) *Œstrin*, which induces "heat" (pro-œstrum and œstrus). This substance has now been produced in crystalline form, and appears to be effective when taken orally on an empty stomach.

According to Bellerby ("Medical Problems of Contraception," *Brit. Med. Journ.*, May 28th, 1932, p. 1000) injection of œstrin prevents embedding of the ovum, but it does not prevent fertilisation. In an early stage of pregnancy it would produce reabsorption; in a later stage it would be abortifacient.

Early reabsorption of the embryo is known to occur in mammals, as a result of lethal genes: it can be produced in animals by diet.

(*b*) *Lutein or progestin*, necessary for the maintenance of pregnancy. This hormone promotes the raised nutrition of the uterus and the growth of the mammary glands in preparation for lactation. It is elaborated during the luteal phase of the ovarian cycle.

(*c*) There is probably a third hormone which is responsible for the growth of the female secondary sex characters.

Testicular Hormone

Proviron, which appears to be responsible for the secondary male characters.

Pituitary Sex Hormones

The anterior lobe of the pituitary produces:—

(*a*) *An œstrogenic hormone*, which acts also on the male organs.

(*b*) *A lutealising hormone.* A functional correlation exists between these pituitary sex hormones and the ovarian hormones. The gonads are inactive in the absence of the anterior lobe of the pituitary; and a physiological antagonism between the internal secretion of the posterior pituitary and the secretion of the corpus luteum has been demonstrated.

Bellerby reports the success of his experimental work on the termination of pregnancy in the rabbit by a single intravenous injection of an extract prepared from the anterior lobe of the pituitary (*Journal of Experimental Biology*, July, 1935). The injection induced ovulation in *pregnant* rabbits, and this was almost invariably associated with resorption or abortion of the embryo. He suggests that this termination of pregnancy may be due either to the direct action of the extract upon the uterus, or to a toxic effect on the embryo, or to the cessation of function of the corpora lutea of pregnancy.

Provided the hormonic control of the reproductive cycle has no secondary ill-effects, and can be regulated to produce a definite temporary sterility in woman, there appears to be some hope that the sex hormones may be utilised for contraceptive purposes in the future. Such a biological method of contraception would be a distinct advance on present methods.

Formation of Spermatoxins

Metchnikoff and other investigators discovered that the injection of spermatozoa into warm-blooded animals results in the formation of spermatoxins. The resulting immunisation was first believed to be specific for the species, but later work showed that immunity can be induced with foreign, dead spermatozoa. It is suggested that the absorption of semen from the human vagina during coitus may diminish fertility, and in certain cases may be the cause of sterility. The possibility of producing a temporary sterility in woman by the injection of human semen is being investigated. Animal experiments on the prevention of conception through spermatoxins are promising; but the experiments on women reported up to the present appear to be inconclusive, chiefly because of the short period of observation and lack of controls.

An investigation of the experimental work on the control of conception by means of spermatoxins, carried out at the Prophylactic

(Birth Control) Clinic of the Regional Scientific Institute for the Protection of Motherhood, in Moscow, made in September, 1933, is reported in the *Journal of Contraception*, December, 1935. The injection fluid is a sterile preparation of ejaculate containing three to five millions of sperms in each cubic centimetre. Injections were given in increasing doses from ½ c.c. up to 5 c.c. at three to four days interval, and a total of twelve to eighteen injections were given. Nursing mothers and women suffering from any inflammatory conditions were excluded from the tests. Treatment was begun in 1932, and thirty-seven women had been immunised. A second course of injections, consisting of only one-half the amount of the first course, is given after an interval of five months. A few of the women had chills and a high temperature with some anaphylactic manifestations; but the menstrual and sexual life of the patients was reported to be unaffected. Two failures are reported.

Naiditch (New Research in Contraceptive Methods—" Temporary Sterility obtained by the Introduction of Spermatozoa," 1928, published by the Commission for the Study of Contraceptive Methods appointed by the Department of Protection of Mother and Child of Soviet Russia) claims 81 per cent. successes in his investigation of the effects of subcutaneous injection of dead bull sperms into healthy fertile women: twenty-six out of the total thirty-two women, in *periods varying from two to twelve months*, did not become pregnant. In the opinion of the writer, it is most probable that a similar percentage of sterility would be obtained from a control group of women.

Baskin (*Amer. Journ. Obstet. and Gynæcol.*, December, 1932) has injected human spermatic fluid intramuscularly. The resultant marked spermicidal properties in the blood serum gradually diminished until, at the end of twelve months, the serum failed to kill spermatozoa. The cervical secretions were non-spermicidal at all times. None of the patients became pregnant within twelve months; and re-vaccination at the end of the year appeared to renew the immunity for at least twelve months. In a later communication (*Journal of Contraception*, December, 1935) he reports: " At the present time we have records of over one hundred women immunised. The dosage varied, but usually consisted of four injections at five to seven day intervals as follows: 2 c.c., 8 c.c., 10 c.c., 10 c.c. The material injected consists of animal spermatozoa in Ringer's solution, to which Merthiolate had been added as an antiseptic and Chloretone as a preservative. The injections are given intramuscularly into the buttocks. The dosage will probably have to be adjusted in individual cases. We have been able to immunise all our patients, although some have received more injections when we were unable to demonstrate a marked immunity after the four injections. The average immunity persists for about one year, but one case became pregnant in six months. No effects on the well-being, blood, menses, or sexual reactions have been observed. . . . We have immunised women and kept them sterile for six years by yearly injections."

It is too early to say whether such a serological method of inducing a temporary sterility is likely to be of practical use in human contraception. *As in the case of hormonic sterility, the conditions of reliability, harmlessness and definite control of the period of temporary sterility must be fulfilled.*

Conclusion

Meanwhile, since advice on methods of contraception for securing the greatest possible protection against pregnancy involves a consideration of the following :—

i. Direct ejaculation of semen into the cervical os, or even into the cervical canal in some cases, may occur.

ii. Spermatozoa within the vagina are protected from the action of chemical spermicides by the alkaline cervical mucus, the mucus plug (Kristeller) at the cervical os, and to a certain extent by the seminal fluid itself.

iii. Some of the millions of motile spermatozoa in the ejaculate may find their way into crevices within the vaginal mucous membrane which have proved inaccessible to spermicides, even to those of the foaming variety or to those administered by a douche.

iv. Living motile spermatozoa may be present within the vagina for an unknown period—certainly for several hours—following coitus.

v. We cannot determine definitely, for any particular patient, at what period, if any, in her menstrual cycle she is physiologically sterile. This problem is further complicated by the possibility of irregular ovulation due to the influence of hormones, etc.

we may draw the following conclusions :—

1. Contraceptive measures on every occasion of coitus are advisable.

2. A combination of mechanical and chemical methods should be recommended, *e.g.*,

(*a*) a mechanical barrier (sheath or occlusive pessary) between the cervix and the ejaculate ; and

(*b*) a chemical spermicide (suppository, tablet, jelly or douche) :—

(i.) to kill spermatozoa within the vagina and so to prevent them from entering the uterus after penetrating the space between the rim of an occlusive pessary, or after the mechanical barrier has been removed ;

(ii.) to compensate to some extent for any imperfections of occlusive pessaries or sheaths—such as a flaw or tear in the rubber ; and

(iii.) to provide as far as possible an additional barrier between the rim of a pessary and the vaginal or cervical tissue.

Note.—The object of using an occlusive pessary is not, as has been suggested in criticism, to make it impossible for spermatozoa to reach the os. To attempt by mechanical obstruction to block their progress along the moist mucous membrane towards the cervix would involve painful and exceedingly harmful pressure of the local tissues, and would doubtless be quite futile. The space between the vaginal or cervical tissues and the rim of the most perfect fitting occlusive pessary is so extensive in relation to the microscopic sperm that there is no physical obstruction to the passage of sperms along the vaginal or cervical mucous membrane in this region. An attempt to diminish or obliterate this space is made by lubricating the rim of the occlusive pessary with a spermicidal ointment or jelly ; but it is unlikely that sufficient of the lubricant remains on the rim, when the pessary has been adjusted, to form a sperm-proof joint. It is hoped that the spermicides used below the cap may have time to immobilise or kill the sperms in the ejaculate before they can pass the mechanical barrier ; and a further supply of spermicide—such as the spermicidal lubricant of the cap—placed above the cap acts as an additional safeguard. *The purpose of an occlusive pessary is to prevent the ejaculate from being deposited on or in the region of the cervix, and particularly to prevent direct ejaculation into a dilated os in those cases in which this would be possible.* In addition, the occlusive appliance, by confining the ejaculate to the vagina out of contact with the cervix, facilitates the effectiveness of the chemical spermicide on account of the time factor.

CHAPTER III

METHODS OF CONTRACEPTION

CHEMICAL CONTRACEPTIVES

General Considerations.—In recent years great progress has been made in the knowledge of the spermicidal power of various chemical substances. To-day we know that a good germicide is not necessarily a good spermicide, and we recognise that the efficacy of spermicidal preparations depends upon at least two factors :—

(*a*) the chemical or spermicide ;
(*b*) the vehicle.

We must bear in mind that a high spermicidal power of a substance does not necessarily mean that it is a correspondingly effective constituent of a suppository, foam tablet, jelly or douche, or even that it is at all suitable for this purpose. Reactions *in vitro* may vary considerably from those *in vivo*. For instance, a vehicle containing a high percentage of glycerine will have a dehydrating effect on the tissues, and consequently dilution of the spermicide with serous exudate will result. Dilution by normal vaginal secretions and by the seminal fluid, and, in the case of acids, the buffering or protective action of the seminal fluid are also important factors to be considered. When the practical difficulties of effective mixing with a suitable vehicle have been overcome, and the resultant preparation has been shown to be harmless and non-irritating to the local tissues, the final evaluation must rest upon clinical results.

However effective the combination of chemical and vehicle, and however effective its distribution in the vagina, it may fail in its purpose if the ejaculate passes directly into the cervical canal. Until this possibility can be definitely eliminated, the greatest possible protection against pregnancy still involves the additional use of a mechanical barrier to protect the cervix from contact with the ejaculate.

Desirable Characteristics of Chemical Contraceptives

It is possible that no single form of chemical contraceptive will prove generally acceptable, on account of variations in economic status, frequency of coitus, climatic conditions and personal idiosyncrasies. The use of apparatus, however simple, for inserting jellies or for douching; the "messiness" of suppositories or jellies; the irritation caused to the vaginal mucous membrane or to the penis; the inconvenience of douching; the failure of foam tablets to dissolve —these are some of the objections likely to be met with in contraceptive practice. It is the writer's experience that ninety-nine patients may be using a particular chemical contraceptive without the least discomfort, and the hundredth may experience vaginal irritation from its use.

The following characteristics of a chemical contraceptive are desirable :—

1. It should be harmless if absorbed from the vagina into the blood-stream.
2. It should be non-irritant to the vagina, uterus and penis.
3. It should not disturb the normal vaginal flora.
4. It should be incapable of causing genetic modification of sperms which may survive a sublethal dose and retain their fertilising power.
5. It should be within the patient's economic means. Frequency of coitus has a bearing on contraceptive costs.
6. It should be easy to use.
7. It should be æsthetically unobjectionable—no unpleasant odour, non-staining, small in bulk, and its mode of application acceptable.
8. It should be harmless to rubber, so that it may be used in conjunction with an occlusive pessary or washable sheath.
9. It should have optimum viscosity to secure adhesion to vaginal and cervical surfaces.
10. It should have good spreading power, and therefore should have a low surface tension to facilitate distribution into all the vaginal rugæ.
11. It should have a high spermicidal power, with a

wide margin of safety. According to Baker,[1] it is desirable that the spermicide should be eight times as powerful as is necessary to kill all sperms in laboratory experiments.

12. Its spermicidal action should be effective within the range of vaginal acidity or alkalinity.

13. It should be unaffected by the range of temperature to which it may be subjected. Suppositories which have a low melting point are unsuitable for the tropics.

Since many patients do, in fact, rely upon the use of a chemical contraceptive without the additional safeguard of a mechanical barrier, I regard the *time factor* as of great importance. The shorter the time taken to kill all the spermatozoa the better; therefore it is desirable that a spermicidal preparation should fulfil the remaining conditions of harmlessness and general suitability and should act practically instantaneously.

A spermicide which is also a good germicide and which would be effective in the prevention and cure of venereal and other infections, would have particular value.

An investigation of the *spermicidal* powers of certain chemicals has been carried out by Dr. John R. Baker, under the auspices of the Birth Control Investigation Committee.

Baker devised a technique for determining the least concentration—which he calls the immobilising concentration—of any substance, in the series 2 per cent., 1 per cent., $\frac{1}{2}$ per cent., $\frac{1}{4}$ per cent., $\frac{1}{8}$ per cent., $\frac{1}{16}$ per cent., $\frac{1}{32}$ per cent., etc., which will completely immobilise all sperms in half an hour at 37° C. in four consecutive experiments, the control sperms showing normal activity. In evaluating the spermicidal powers of chemicals, I am adopting his findings.

The highest activity is 3+, complete immobility is 0, and diminishing grades of activity 3, 2+, 2, 1+, 1.

He is using cavy sperms as the experimental animal, for he has found that they closely resemble human sperms in their reactions to the most diverse substances; moreover, the sperms are large and very active and adequate supplies

[1] "Chemical Control of Conception" (Chapman and Hall, 1935).

are available. He has elaborated suitable suspension fluids for keeping mammalian sperms at maximum activity at body temperature :—

Buffered glucose-saline (B.G.S.), with a *p*H 8·1, for testing direct action of substances on sperms.

Acetate glucose-saline (A.G.S.), for the salts of metals whose phosphates are insoluble.

Albumen-saline, for imitating the protective action of semen on sperms.

Phosphate-albumen, for testing spermicidal power of acids.

Lactic saline, for testing substances in slightly acid environment.

The following lists bring out clearly the marked differences in the germicidal and spermicidal powers of certain substances, and also the great variations in their spermicidal powers. It will be seen also that certain substances which are used for their spermicidal properties in some proprietary chemical contraceptives are relatively weak spermicides. I must emphasise, however, that before any substance can be recommended for contraceptive purposes, it must be capable of combination with a suitable base, and this combination must be stable, harmless in use, and otherwise unobjectionable.

Pure Substances Graded according to Spermicidal Power with Cavy Sperms in B.G.S. or A.G.S.[1]

I.C. represents the immobilising concentration tested by Baker's technique.

Grade 9. *I.C.* $\frac{1}{512}$ *per cent.* :—
Toluquinone.
Butylquinone.
Methoxyquinone.
Ethylquinone.
Parabenzoquinone.
Paraxyloquinone.

Grade 8. *I.C.* $\frac{1}{256}$ *per cent.* :—
Mercuric chloride.
Methoxyhydroquinone.
Formaldehyde.
Paraformaldehyde.
Methylhydroquinone.

Grade 7. *I.C.* $\frac{1}{128}$ *per cent.* :—
Malachite green.
Thymoquinone.
Butylhydroquinone.

Grade 6. *I.C.* $\frac{1}{64}$ *per cent.* :—
Saponine.
Methoxytoluquinone.
Hexylresorcin.
Dimethoxyhydroquinone.
Oxyhydroquinone.
Iodine (with four times as much potassium iodide).
Orthoethoxysalicylaldehyde.

1 "Chemical Control of Conception," by John R. Baker, M.A., D.Phil. (Chapman and Hall, 1935).

Orthovanillin.
Hydroquinone.

Grade 5. *I.C.* $\frac{1}{32}$ *per cent.* :—
Salicylaldehyde.
Crystal violet.
Thymol.
Sodium oleate.
Sodium palmitate.

Grade 4. *I.C.* $\frac{1}{16}$ *per cent.* :—
Potassium permanganate.
Ethylharmol hydrochloride.

Grade 3. *I.C.* $\frac{1}{8}$ *per cent.* :—
Mercurochrome.
Carmine (with four times as much borax).
Harmine hydrochloride.

Grade 2. *I.C.* $\frac{1}{4}$ *per cent.* :—
Sodium taurocholeate.
Zinc sulphate.
Potassium aluminium sulphate —anhydrous.
Sodium glycocholeate.
Dioxyquinoline sulphate.
Quinine urea hydrochloride.
Chinosol.
Cresol.
Potassium borotartrate.

Grade 1. *I.C.* $\frac{1}{2}$ *per cent.* :—
Quinine hydrochloride.
Potassium oxyquinoline sulphonate.
Potassium cyanide.
Quinine bisulphate.
Catechol.
Phenol.

Grade 0. *I.C.* 1 *per cent.* :—
Hydroquinone methyl ether.
Acetaldehyde.
Chloral hydrate.
Resorcinol.

Grade −1. *I.C.* 2 *per cent.* :—
Pyrogallol.
Potassium capronate.
Orthophenylene diamine.

Ungraded. These fail to immobilise at 2 *per cent.* :—
Ammonium chloride.
Zinc sulphocarbolate.
Potassium butyrate.
Sodium citrate.
Hexamine.
Sodium tartrate.
Magnesium sulphate.
Borax.
Ethyl alcohol.
Metaphenylene diamine.
Glycerol.
Sodium dichlorylsulphaminobenzoate.

Standard Test of Pure Substances with Cavy Sperms in Albumen Saline [1]

Note.—Baker states that cavy sperms suspended in albumen-saline behave almost exactly like human sperms in human semen. Albumen-saline is used when testing the spermicidal power of substances in the presence of a protein protector.

Grade 8. *I.C.* $\frac{1}{256}$ *per cent.* :—
Toluquinone.
Methylhydroquinone.
Ethylhydroquinone.

Grade 6. *I.C.* $\frac{1}{64}$ *per cent.* :—
Hexylresorcinol.

Grade 3. *I.C.* $\frac{1}{8}$ *per cent.* :—
Mercuric chloride.
Normal propylresorcinol.
Orthovanillin.

Grade 1. *I.C.* $\frac{1}{2}$ *per cent.* :—
Sodium oleate.
Chinosol.

Grade 0. *I.C.* 1 *per cent.* :—
Zinc sulphate.
Methylhydroquinone (with twice as much anhydrous sodium sulphite).

Grade −1. *I.C.* 2 *per cent.* :—
Potassium borotartrate.

Ungraded. These fail to immobilise at 2 *per cent.* :—
Sodium sulphite.
Borax.

[1] "Chemical Control of Conception," by John R. Baker, M.A., D.Phil. (Chapman and Hall, 1935).

Acids.—The spermicidal power of acids depends upon *p*H—the extent to which they ionise ; the anion appears to be much less important.

Baker found that

Below *p*H 5·0—all sperms were immobilised.
At *p*H 5·0 to 5·9—less than 10 per cent. were moderately active.
At *p*H 6·0 to 6·9—less than half were moderately active.

Note.—*p*H represents the unit of degree of acidity or alkalinity :—

neutral —*p*H 7,
alkaline —greater than *p*H 7,
acid —less than *p*H 7.

There is a possibility that acids may immobilise sperms without killing them, except at a *p*H of 3·5 or lower.

According to Baker, it is the concentration of hydrogen ions, and not the nature of the anions, that determines the inactivity of the sperms. It makes little difference what acid is used ; all have much the same effect at the same *p*H. The *rate of dissociation* may produce apparent exceptions to this rule, as in the case of boric acid, which, being a very weak acid, kills only at such high concentrations that osmotic pressure is probably concerned in its action.

Another important factor which affects the spermicidal power of acids is their ability to overcome the alkaline buffer of the semen or suspension fluid ; thus the suspension fluid for testing acids should have the same alkaline reserve as human semen. Baker finds that acids are weak spermicides in the presence of semen :—

Grade 1.	Acetic acid. Sulphuric acid.	*K.C.* ½ *per cent.*
Grade 2.	Succinic. Tartaric. Citric.	*K.C.* 1 *per cent.*

The *normal* vaginal fluid is slightly acid in reaction (*p*H 4·45 to 3·86). Döderlein's bacillus, which has its habitat in the vagina, produces lactic acid. The secretion of the cervical glands is normally alkaline, and pathological secretions are also alkaline. Little is known of the normal variations in vaginal acidity during the menstrual cycle.

During sexual excitement the quantity of vaginal fluid is greatly increased by the neutral or alkaline secretions of the cervix (1 to 4 c.c.). The *p*H of the vaginal contents will be still further raised by the addition of the alkaline semen (about 5 c.c.). The alkalinity must be neutralised before acids can exert their spermicidal action. The presence of buffers diminishes the power of any substance to affect the *p*H of a solution ; and the protein content of the semen has a buffering effect. Acids in a cocoa-butter or greasy ointment base do not ionise owing to the absence of water ; the spermicidal power of such preparations is therefore very weak or entirely absent unless other spermicides which act independently of ionisation are incorporated.

Lactic Acid.—This is used in suppositories, tablets, jellies, ointments, and douches. A contraceptive jelly (" Biolactine ") containing a culture of lactic acid-forming organisms has been introduced in Germany and Russia.[1] Its use as a contraceptive was favoured because lactic acid is normally present, at a concentration of about 0·5 per cent., in the vaginal fluid. According to Moench, sperms live for hours in a 0·5 per cent. solution of lactic acid, and a 1 per cent. solution takes three hours to immobilise all the sperms. It is a weak spermicide.

Jellies and ointments, which depend upon lactic acid alone for their spermicidal effect, contain from 1·5 to 2 per cent. of lactic acid. Anything over 1·5 per cent., however, causes smarting of the vaginal mucous membrane in a number of cases, while some few patients cannot tolerate even 1·5 per cent., which may be regarded as the lowest effective strength. For such people lactic acid alone in a vehicle is unsuitable. Some lactic acid ointments are quite ineffective as spermicides, as lactates are formed, giving the ointment an alkaline reaction.

[1] For details see "The Contraceptive and Curative Effect of 'Biolactine,'" Dr. Y. C. Dubintschnik, Fifth Report of International Group for the Investigation of Contraception, 1934 (National Birth Control Association).

The strength of the solution for a douche is 1 drachm to the quart.

Acetic acid is commonly used, in the form of dilutions of vinegar, as a post-coital douche (an ounce to the quart) and for medicating sponges or tampons (2 ounces to the cupful).

Citric acid, in the form of lemon juice, is used in the same way as acetic acid. Two tablespoonfuls of lemon juice to a quart of water gives a suitable strength for a douche. Citric acid is a constituent of " G.P." ointment and " G.P." solubles.

Boric acid is a very weak spermicide ; it has some value as a preservative. It is used in contraceptive jellies, ointments, suppositories, and tablets.

Carbonic acid, produced by the interaction of acids and sodium bicarbonate, is formed in most foaming mixtures. It is an unstable acid which liberates the inert gas carbon dioxide. This gas may be lethal to spermatozoa, although the immobilisation of sperms in the seminal vesicles by expired CO_2 and the subsequent activation by the prostatic secretion suggests that a high concentration is required to kill. However, it certainly immobilises them. Carbonic acid is, therefore, a useful vehicle on account of its mechanical action in producing a foam ; and it may increase the spermicidal power of the foaming mixture on account of the carbon dioxide evolved.

Carbolic acid (phenol) has been shown by Baker to be a relatively *weak spermicide.* Its intensely poisonous nature, and its tendency to be absorbed by mucous membranes and by wound surfaces, contra-indicates its use as a spermicide, either as a douche or in any other form.

Cresylic acid (cresol) is only a little less dangerous than carbolic acid, and only slightly more spermicidal. The various cresol preparations, including the emulsion *Lysol,* which is commonly used in the form of a douche, are best discarded in favour of substances which are equally or more spermicidal and which are entirely non-toxic.

The low *p*H (2·9) of Mil-San jelly is obtained by the inclusion of a combination of acids (acetic, lactic, boric, tartaric and formic) in weak concentration.

Other Substances.—*Alum* (potassium aluminium sulphate) has an immobilising concentration of $\frac{1}{4}$ per cent., and is therefore a moderate spermicide. It is largely used as a therapeutic agent for its astringent properties. Dilute solutions have an astringent action on mucous membranes, while concentrated solutions and alum in powder form act as irritants. For contraceptive purposes it is used as a douche, in powder form, and as a constituent of jellies and tablets. An alum douche (1 drachm to the pint) is used in cases of relaxed vagina or of leucorrhœa.

Chinosol is only slightly more spermicidal than the salts of quinine (I.C. $\frac{1}{4}$ per cent.), and is therefore a relatively weak spermicide. Carleton's experimental work on rabbits and bitches indicates that it is comparatively innocuous. It is used in some suppositories, foam tablets and jellies.

Formaldehyde in watery solution (formalin) proves to be as strongly spermicidal as corrosive sublimate, and it is non-toxic and non-irritating in very much greater concentrations than the killing concentration, which is $\frac{1}{256}$.

Carleton found that it did not injure the vagina or uterus of the rabbit in concentrations " far greater than the killing concentration."

Baker suggests a weak solution of formalin as a vaginal douche, and remarks " one cannot detect formaldehyde if a solution at the killing concentration is taken into the mouth and swallowed. The preparation of a solid pessary containing or producing formaldehyde presents difficulties. . . ." It is a constituent of " G.P." ointment (Gilmont Products).

Hexamine produces formaldehyde only very slowly, and is, consequently, a very weak spermicide (killing concentration greater than 2 per cent.).

Hexylresorcin, with a killing concentration $\frac{1}{64}$ per cent., ranks high as a spermicide. In addition, it has in solution a low surface tension, which facilitates its effective distribution into the crevices of the vaginal mucous membrane, and it acts in either acid or alkaline medium. It is prescribed internally as caprokol in doses of 5–15 gm. t.d.s. as a urinary antiseptic, and it is used as a douche for leucorrhœa. Its harmlessness, when it is used as a spermicide, has been determined clinically. It is a constituent of "G.P." jelly, PermFoam jelly, Prentif jelly, Prensols and Prentif suppositories.

Iodine (dissolved with four times its weight of potassium iodide) has a killing concentration of $\frac{1}{64}$ per cent.

It is used in the form of a post-coital douche (1 drachm to the pint).

According to Konikow ("Physicians' Manual of Birth Control," p. 114), the intra-uterine application of iodine has been used extensively in Germany and Russia as a method of contraception. Iodine (a 10 per cent. solution or equal parts of iodine and glycerine) is injected into the uterus, or is used for swabbing the uterine cavity, once a month before menstruation, or a few days after its delay. The chemical is used, not for its immediate spermicidal action, but for its local effect on the endometrium, to prevent the nidation of a fertilised ovum or to destroy an early embedded ovum. As may be expected, the results are disastrous in many cases, and deaths are reported.

This method is now condemned by Selitzky of the Moscow State Hospital (Contraceptive Methods in the Light of Modern Science, State Department of Health, Moscow, 1929).

Mercuric chloride (corrosive sublimate), although a powerful spermicide (killing concentration $\frac{1}{256}$ per cent.), is definitely contra-indicated for contraceptive purposes on account of its intensely poisonous nature. Several deaths are recorded from its use in solution as a douche and in tablet form inserted into the vagina.

Methylhydroquinone (immobilising concentration $\frac{1}{256}$ per cent.) is a very strong spermicide. A 1 per cent. suspension in the fat base cocola was found by Carleton to be harmless when inserted per vaginum in rabbits and bitches, but proved an irritant when injected in solution in normal saline. According to Baker, however, it turns semen brown, and is less spermicidal in the presence of acids.

Potassium permanganate acts as a protoplasmic poison by oxidising proteins; it liberates oxygen in the presence of organic matter. As a spermicide its immobilising concentration in B.G.S. is $\frac{1}{16}$ per cent. but, according to Baker, few sperms remain alive at half that concentration. He suggests that it interferes with the respiration of the sperms. It is used chiefly as a douche (1 in 2,000, or $\frac{1}{20}$ per cent.).

Quinine has probably been more widely used for contraceptive purposes during the past fifty years than any other drugs. Quinine and the allied alkaloids are used in douches, ointments, jellies, tablets, suppositories, medicated oils and in powder form. The work of Baker, Voge and others has shown that quinine is a *relatively poor spermicide;* the hydrochloride and bisulphate have an immobilising concentration of $\frac{1}{2}$ per cent., and the urea hydrochloride is only slightly more spermicidal. The relative clinical success of cocoa-butter suppositories containing quinine is probably due largely to the mechanical barrier formed by the vehicle, and, in the case of Rendell's pessaries, to the acidity.

A further reason for the abandonment of quinine as a contraceptive is its potential harmfulness. There is ample clinical evidence that quinine in the vagina may cause local irritation, and that its vaginal absorption into the bloodstream may cause severe toxic symptoms. Cases have been recorded of the development of specific toxic symptoms (tinnitus, headaches, giddiness) after the use of soluble suppositories containing quinine by patients who are hypersensitive to the drug; and such allergic effects as urticaria, dermatitis and collapse have been recorded. Booysen ("Quinine as a Contraceptive," *Marriage Hygiene*, Vol. II, No. I, August, 1935) relates that ten of twenty-seven consecutive clinic patients using quinine suppositories complained of vaginal irritation, and she has observed a few cases of cervical erosions which have appeared following the use of quinine urea hydrochloride tablets and which disappeared with no other treatment than cessation of their use. One case of severe ulceration with purulent discharge is reported. These findings of local trauma have been confirmed in the writer's clinical experience, and are supported by the experimental work of Carleton and Florey (chapter on the Pathology of Contraception in "The Chemical Control of Conception," Chapman and Hall, 1935), who found that quinine urea hydrochloride induced necrosis and sloughing of the endometrium when injected into the uterus of the laboratory animals, and that repeated daily vaginal injections of a solution of this salt in bitches caused marked vaginitis with areas of ulceration. Suppositories containing quinine in cocoa-butter, however, were found to be harmless, the slight desquamation of the superficial layers of the vaginal mucous membrane being regarded by Carleton as probably within physiological limits.

Although idiosyncrasies to quinine may be rare, yet in view of its relatively weak spermicidal power, and of the possibility of harmful local and constitutional effects, the use of quinine as a contraceptive should be abandoned in favour of other substances which are much more effective spermicides and which have proved experimentally quite harmless, even to the delicate epithelium of the rabbit.

Soaps.—Sodium oleate and sodium palmitate, tested with human sperms in human semen, have a killing concentration of ½ per cent., a spermicidal power equal to that of quinine and chinosol. They are surface tension depressants, and have therefore good spreading power. According to Voge, however, the spermicidal power of a soap solution depends upon the degree of emulsification attained. He found that "with 1 per cent. solution added to semen it took three times the volume of soap to semen to act promptly and emulsification was essential, as mere contact did not produce any result." It would appear, therefore, that the seminal fluid needs to be thoroughly mixed with the soapy solution for an effective spermicidal effect to be achieved; otherwise the raised *p*H of the hydrolised soap solution (*p*H 8·5–9·5, or slightly alkaline) would be a disadvantage.

The free alkali of a soapy solution may irritate mucous membranes, the degree of irritation depending upon the amount of free alkali present. Carleton [1] found that "concentrations of 8 per cent. to 25 per cent. of sodium oleate in cocola caused an intense vaginitis, with patchy necrosis and desquamation of the mucosa, after seven or more daily injections" per vaginum in bitches. Clinically, I have had no evidence of irritation or injury due to the use of a soapy

[1] "The Chemical Control of Conception," by John R. Baker, M.A. D.Phil. (Chapman and Hall, 1935).

water douche or to the lubrication of an occlusive pessary with soap solution. Nevertheless, rare cases of vaginitis due to the use of soap or soap flakes containing free soda have been reported. Thousands of clinic patients have for periods of years regularly used the soapy douche without apparent harm ; and recently I saw a patient, æt. 36, with three children born at intervals of two years, who subsequently, on the advice of her doctor, had relied successfully for a period of eight years on the use of a piece of soap about the size of a hazel nut as a vaginal suppository before coitus, which occurred on an average twice a week. She had no signs or symptoms of local irritation or injury, and, on examination with a speculum, I found the vagina and cervix quite healthy in appearance.

The popularity of the soapy douche as a contraceptive measure is probably due to its cheapness and accessibility. The process of douching brings about good emulsification and mixing with semen, so there is no reason to doubt its efficacy as a spermicide. It is probably wise to advise limiting its use to not more than twice a week, and to warn patients against the use of unsuitable soaps, such as the cheap household soaps and soap flakes which contain free alkali.

About $\frac{3}{5}$ ounce of soap to a quart of water gives approximately a 1 per cent. solution. The syringe needs to be rinsed in clear water after use.

As emergency measures, intra-vaginal lathering, or the use of certain shaving creams and dentifrices has been suggested. However, the presence of irritants in the latter precludes their regular use ; and the high concentration of soap produced by lathering would almost certainly be injurious. These methods are not to be recommended.

Toluquinone, the most spermicidal substance known, has an immobilising concentration of $\frac{1}{512}$ per cent. Its use clinically as a contraceptive is precluded by its harmfulness, as Carleton found that it caused a vaginitis in experimental animals.

Water immobilises sperms rapidly, and, according to Steinhauser, they are killed in ten seconds by ordinary tap-water.

It is pointed out by Dickinson and Bryant, however,

that in order to kill sperms instantly, a *mixture* of semen and water in the proportion of one (semen) to three (water) is necessary. "No such quantity," they remark, "will stay within the vagina."—("Control of Conception," p. 45.)

A post-coital *douche* of plain water, however, may be effective in dealing with any living sperms in the vagina, provided that no salts, which have been used as a contraceptive before douching, dissolve into the water. Such a solution would no longer immunise sperms unless the salt were in spermicidal strength.

Zinc sulphate has a killing concentration equal to that of alum (¼ per cent.). It is occasionally prescribed in solution as an astringent and disinfectant douche in cases of leucorrhœa.

The *sulphocarbolate*, a constituent of two of the foam tablets, is a very weak spermicide, failing to kill at 2 per cent. (Baker).

Vehicles.—The vehicle or carrier of the spermicide is used primarily for its mechanical action, and this mechanical action is an important factor in the efficacy of the chemical contraceptive. Vehicles in use include the following :—

Cocoa-butter Cocola Gelatine	for suppositories.
Glycerine Glycerite of starch Gum acacia (arabic) Gum tragacanth Agar-agar Irish moss	for jellies, pastes and ointments, and foam preparations.
Foam producing substances (sodium bicarbonate with acids). Colloids (*e.g.*, gelatine or egg albumen).	for foaming tablets and foaming jellies.
Olive oil.	

Cocoa-butter is a vegetable fat with an odour which proves disagreeable to most patients. Odourless and scented preparations are now made. Cocoa-butter has a melting point well below body heat (91·4° F.); adulterants, such as white wax, are sometimes added to raise the melting point of cocoa-butter suppositories which are to be used in hot climates. It is used as a vehicle for suppositories containing quinine, lactic acid, chinosol, etc. In some cases cocoa-butter pessaries fail to melt at body temperature, or they melt too slowly.

Cocoa-butter injures rubber; it should not be used in contact with a rubber pessary or a washable sheath.

Baker has disproved the idea, formerly held, that cocoa-butter inhibits the movements of sperms. There is ample clinical evidence, however, that cocoa-butter suppositories are, in fact, moderately good contraceptives. It is possible that the cocoa-butter acts by forming a mechanical barrier of oily film, analogous to the rubber occlusive pessary.

Cocola, a proprietary product of secret composition, is a fat which is used to replace cocoa-butter in suppositories. It is almost odourless. As it has an actively deleterious effect on rubber, cocola suppositories should not be used in combination with a rubber pessary or with a washable sheath.

In his earlier experiments, with suppositories provided by manufacturers, Baker found cocola superior to cocoa-butter as a vehicle for chinosol and quinine; and his findings were announced in the medical press. However, he has more recently made 4 per cent. suspensions of chinosol in cocola and in cocoa-butter for himself, and the spermicidal powers of these are the same. It is possible that the cocoa-butter suppositories provided by the manufacturers contained much less chinosol than they thought. Cocoa-butter does not prevent the action of chinosol on sperms.

Gelatine is a protein which, in dilute watery solution, forms a gel with a melting point at body temperature. Although devoid of the messiness and unpleasant odour of cocoa-butter, it has not the mechanical contraceptive action of the vegetable fat; but in spite of the buffering action of gelatine, spermicides in a gelatine base produce their maximum effect in about half the time required for the same spermicides in a cocoa-butter base. Gelatine is commonly used as a vehicle for spermicides in suppositories and jellies.

Glycerine, the alcohol glycerol, is a decomposition product of animal or vegetable fats and fixed oils. It is completely soluble in water, and acts as a solvent for a number of drugs. It is used in contraceptive ointments and jellies and suppositories, as a solvent for other substances, and also to produce a suitable viscosity. Its powerful dehydrating action on mucous membranes, which may cause severe smarting, renders it unsuitable for full-strength use in the vagina; and the consequent dilution of the spermicide with the serous exudate is a further drawback to its use except in weak concentration.

Glycerite of starch, a jelly formed by heating starch with water and glycerine, is used as a component of contraceptive jellies, suppositories and tablets. Too great a proportion of this compound may liberate an excessive amount of glycerine in the vagina.

Gums (gum arabic and gum tragacanth) are carbohydrates closely related to starch.

Gum arabic (acacia) is composed of salts of arabinic acid. Its acid content has a spermicidal value. It is soluble in water and is used as a vehicle for other drugs. Gum tragacanth contains salts of arabin and tragacanthin. In water it is insoluble, but swells up into a jelly.

Agar-agar is a carbohydrate obtained from various East Indian seaweeds. Like tragacanth, it is insoluble in water, but swells up into a jelly.

Irish moss is incompatible with acids. It swells up in water to form a mucilage.

Foam-producing Substances.—Sodium bicarbonate in combination with acids (tartaric, boric or citric) produces effervescence in the presence of moisture. This base is incorporated with spermicides, colloids, and other substances to form tablets or jellies which, in the presence of sufficient moisture in the case of tablets, form a foam of bubbles of carbon dioxide. The possible advantages of contraceptive foaming preparations are :—

(*a*) The more effective distribution throughout the vagina, provided that, in the case of tablets, there is sufficient moisture in the vagina to effect complete disintegration, and that sufficient bulk of foam is produced in relation to the vaginal cavity. The foaming jelly is independent of vaginal moisture.

(*b*) The action of carbon dioxide, which immobolises sperms. Such foaming mixtures, devoid of other chemicals, have a killing concentration of 8 per cent.

(*c*) The formation of a mechanical barrier of foam.

The *foam tablets* dissolve only in the presence of sufficient moisture, and the vaginal secretions may be markedly deficient ; they require at least three minutes to dissolve. On the other hand, the *foaming jellies* are independent of time or of vaginal moisture, and are thus immediately effective.

Note.—Vaseline and certain greasy substances have an injurious action on gasoline rubber, and should not be allowed to come into contact with rubber pessaries or with rubber condoms which are to be used more than once. They are therefore unsuitable as a vehicle for spermicides to be used in combination with rubber appliances. *Non-greasy* ointments and jellies, and suppositories with a *gelatine* base, should be selected for use in combination with rubber occlusive pessaries and with washable sheaths.

TYPES OF CHEMICAL CONTRACEPTIVES

Suppositories.—Suppositories contain spermicidal chemicals in a solid vehicle which has a melting point at or below body heat. The spermicides in use in proprietary products include aluminium acetotartrate, chinosol, quinine, hexylresorcinol, formaldehyde, salicylic acid, saponin (non-toxic), mercury, lactic acid, boric acid and citric acid.

Method of Use.

1. The suppository should be placed in the upper part of the vagina, as near the cervix as possible, and preferably *after* an occlusive pessary has been adjusted (unless a condom is to be used).

2. Sufficient time before coitus must be allowed for melting (about five minutes); but not longer than ten minutes, in case the solution escapes from the vagina before coitus, unless, of course, the suppository is used *above* a sponge or occlusive pessary.

Suppositories have certain disadvantages. They require that coitus shall be definitely timed so as to take place when the suppository is melted and before it has escaped from the vagina. The act of insertion is an unæsthetic interruption, which for many people spoils the pre-coital "atmosphere." The smell and messiness of the ordinary cocoa-butter group of suppositories are objectionable, and the gelatine suppositories may cause excessive moistness in the vagina.

On the other hand, they have the merit of simplicity and convenience in use.

In patients of known low fertility suppositories alone *may* prove effective. To patients of normal fertility, or in cases where the greatest possible protection against pregnancy is desired, *they should be recommended for use only in conjunction with a mechanical barrier* (pessary or condom). A base of gelatine or some other non-greasy substance should be selected for use in conjunction with a rubber appliance.

Some Proprietary Suppositories [1]

Cocoa-butter Base.

Chinobut (chinosol).
Lam-Butt (quinine).
Martindale's (lactic acid).
Prentif cocoa-butter suppositories (hexylresorcinol and non-toxic saponin).
Proseldis (chinosol).
Quercus (quinine).
Racial (chinosol).
Rendell's (quinine and free acid).

[1] The optimistic claims of the manufacturers and distributors of proprietary contraceptives are frequently unsubstantiated clinically. Moreover, the same chemical contraceptive may cause local irritation in some cases where there is no apparent abnormality of the vaginal mucous membrane, and yet be used with perfect comfort in other cases.

Vimule (quinine).
Waverley (quinine).

Gelatine Base.

Aces (lactic and acetic acids).
Antibion (quinine, boric acid, cresol).
G.P. solubles (citric acid and aluminium aceto-tartras). These are recommended for use with a rubber occlusive pessary only.
Kahm-a-san (boric acid, mercury, salicylic acid).
Lam-Butt (quinine).
Prensols (hexylresorcinol). Large and small sizes.
Prophycols (lactic acid, mercury).
Vimule (quinine).
Wyeth (quinine, boric acid).

Gum Tragacanth and Glycerine.

Docker's Contraps (quinine, lactic acid, magnesium sulphate).

Jellies or Pastes.—These have the advantage of a water-soluble vehicle which facilitates the release of the chemicals. The chemicals are conveyed in a base of combinations of glycerine, glycerite of starch, gums, agar-agar, etc. They act independently of vaginal moisture and of temperature.

They can be used—

(*a*) *As Spermicidal Lubricants for Occlusive Pessaries.*—The whole pessary should be anointed. Many clinic patients prefer ointments for this purpose, because they find the jellies more messy and more apt to flow out of the vagina owing to insufficient viscosity.

(*b*) *For Lubricating the Condom.*—They are eminently suitable for this purpose.

(*c*) *For mass injection into the vagina,* in place of suppository or tablet. They are usually packed in a collapsible tube with a nozzle. A key is sometimes provided to express the jelly from the tube into the upper part of the vagina. Part of the jelly should be expressed into the posterior fornix; the nozzle or tube should then be withdrawn about an inch so that the remainder of the jelly may be expressed just in front of the cervix.

The necessity for cleansing the nozzle after use presents real difficulty in some cases; this difficulty disappears if a number of nozzles is available, each to be used once only and then thrown away. Lead should not be used for the tube or for the nozzle, unless the jelly contains nothing which has a chemical action upon this metal.

The advantage of jellies over tablets or suppositories is that they are ready to act immediately, since they are, as has been previously stated, independent of the variables—time, moisture, pressure and temperature. Accurate timing of coitus is therefore unnecessary. They have the drawback of requiring apparatus for their insertion. In some jellies the viscosity is too low, and they tend to flow out of the vagina prematurely; in others the viscosity is too high, and they do not spread and mix effectively with the seminal fluid.

A jelly which has been extensively prescribed in the past has the formula :—

Lactic acid	1
Boric acid	5
Glycerite of starch, q.s.	ad 100

Chinosol, 0·2 per cent., is added in some instances.

This jelly contains approximately 75 per cent. of glycerine, which would cause the dehydrating effect already referred to under 'Glycerine.' The percentage of boric acid also causes irritation in some cases. Moreover, without the chinosol, the spermicidal power is probably very low.

The large number of proprietary jellies and ointments on the market include the following :—

Antibion (quinine, boric and lactic acids, formates, and an aluminium salt).

Confidol (aluminium acetate, tartaric acid, acetic acid, boracic acid and potassium ortho-oxychinolin-sulphuricum in a vegetable base).

Contraceptalene (lactic and boric acids in a base of glycerite of starch).

Durol (lactic and boric acids, formalin, neutral tragacanth, in base of mel).

Eugam contraceptive jelly (sulphosalicylic acid).
Freelac jelly (lactic and boric acids, glycerine and gum tragacanth).
G.P. jelly (hexylresorcinol, non-toxic saponin, boric acid, vegetable mucilage).
G.P. ointment (citric acid, boric acid, non-toxic saponin, formaldehyde, non-greasy ointment base).
Koromex vaginal jelly (boric, lactic, stearic and the stabiliser).
K.Y. jelly (boric acid in a vegetable base), used as a lubricant.
Mil-San (a number of acids—acetic, lactic, boric, tartaric and formic—with an aluminium compound and chinosol, in a base of tragacanth and glycerine).
Ortho-Gynol jelly (boric acid, oxyquinoline sulphate and glycerine in a vegetable gum base).
Prentif lubricating jelly (hexylresorcinol in a vegetable base).
Prentif compound (quinine and chinosol in a vegetable base).
Proseldis (chinosol, glycerine, gum tragacanth).
Spetonex (ortho-oxycholin sulph. in mucilaginous base).

Mil-San Jelly.—The spermicidal efficacy of this jelly is based on the production of an increase in the natural spermicidal characteristics of the vagina rather than on the use of very powerful spermicides. This effect is secured by the combination of a number of acids in weak concentration so buffered that even with a very low *p*H (2·9) it is claimed that there is no danger of irritation of the mucous membrane.

The action of Mil-San is due to :—

(*a*) An optimum viscosity for promoting adhesion of the jelly to the cervix and vaginal wall. It is claimed that the film of jelly forms a barrier which prevents sperms from reaching the cervical canal before the chemical action of the jelly has immobilised them.

(*b*) A low surface tension, which facilitates a rapid spread of the jelly with penetration into the rugæ of the vaginal surface.

(*c*) Spermicidal properties due to two methods :—

(i.) Agglutination of sperm suspension by the low *p*H and the tri-valent aluminium ion, and

(ii.) Immobilisation of sperms by the several spermicides.

The acidophile bacilli normally present in the healthy vaginal flora are unharmed.

G.P. Ointment is a non-greasy spermicide especially suitable for the lubrication of rubber occlusive pessaries. The base is naturally acid, and the ointment is water-soluble. The melting point is slightly above body temperature, so that the lubricated pessary may be inserted some hours before coitus if desired. Baker finds G.P. ointment to be " the most spermicidal of the ointments studied, both in the test of total spermicidal power and in the diffusion test " (" Chemical Control of Conception," p. 151).

In the selection of suitable cases for the use of jellies, one must bear in mind that the nozzle may cause accidental local trauma, or that the nozzle may be used to penetrate the cervical os in an attempt to procure an abortion. In the large majority of cases, however, especially when the patient has been properly instructed in the use of an occlusive pessary, the risk of accidental injury is probably negligible. Nevertheless, to minimise this risk, a moderately flexible nozzle is preferable to a rigid one, and a bulbous end is desirable. In regard to criminal abortion, if a patient intends to attempt to evacuate the uterus by penetrating the cervical canal, there is no lack of implements among household and toilet objects.

Foaming Preparations.—The primary object of the foaming base is to secure the better distribution of the spermicides ; it has the further advantage that the carbon dioxide in the foam immobilises spermatozoa, provided that ejaculation takes place before the foam breaks down.

1. **Foam Jelly.**—PermFoam is an acid jelly which is contained in a double collapsible tube ; it is packed with a separate tube and nozzle for each application, so that the

need for cleansing the nozzles after use is eliminated. When the tube is compressed the jellies are simultaneously expressed to mix in the nozzle, forming a dense foam charged with carbon dioxide. The foam is expressed into the vagina, and acts independently of temperature and vaginal moisture. The foam has been observed to persist in the vagina for thirty minutes after insertion, and the jelly remains spermicidal within the vagina for at least eight hours after insertion. Two of the constituents, hexylresorcin and saponin (non-toxic), are powerful spermicides and surface tension depressants; moreover, hexylresorcin acts both in an acid and alkaline medium. In addition to being strongly spermicidal, the jelly has the further advantage of being germicidal to pyogenic organisms. It does not deteriorate at extremes of temperature, and should therefore prove to be suitable for use in tropical climates.

Formula of PermFoam

Inner tube containing:	Outer tube containing:
Acid Jelly.	*Bicarbonate Jelly.*
Glycerin amyli.	Glycerin amyli.
Tragacanth.	Tragacanth.
Saponin (non-toxic).	Ovi albumen sicc.
Ac. boric.	Sodium bicarbonate.
Ac. citric.	Hexylresorcinol.
	Aqua ad.

The final foam contains only 10 per cent. of glycerine, and is sufficiently acid to prevent subsequent revitalisation of the spermatozoa.

The *spermicidal power* has been tested by Baker, and compared with the most spermicidal proprietary contraceptive previously tested, and with chinosol (4 per cent.) in cocoa-butter. The results are expressed as the greatest number of cubic centimetres of sperm suspension (guinea-pig sperms in albumen saline, which, according to Baker, gives the same results as human sperms in semen) in which every sperm is killed in three consecutive experiments by 1 gm. of the substance in fifteen minutes.

	1 gram kills all sperms in:
PermFoam. Acid jelly . . .	16 c.c.
The proprietary contraceptive . .	8 ,,
PermFoam. Bicarbonate jelly . .	8 ,,
PermFoam. Complete	4 ,,
Chinosol: 4 per cent. in cocoa-butter .	2 ,,

Since one application of PermFoam is stated to weigh 5·2 gm., it should kill all sperms in approximately 20 c.c. The proprietary contraceptive tablet weighs almost exactly 1 gm., therefore two and a half tablets would equal in spermicidal power the one application of PermFoam.

2. **Foam Tablets.**—Foam tablets contain spermicides in a base—usually bicarbonate of soda and an acid—which, in the presence of sufficient moisture, reacts to form a foam. The effective spermicidal action of the tablets is therefore dependent upon vaginal moisture, and time must be allowed for solution to take place. The foams vary in density, viscosity and stability, according to the ingredients of the foam base.

Disadvantages of foam tablets are :—

(*a*) The satisfactory solution and foam production depend upon an adequacy of vaginal secretion.

In many women, the secretions are deficient, and in such cases the tablet fails to dissolve completely. Some patients find that the tablets dissolve satisfactorily on some occasions, but not on others.

Some manufacturers recommend that the tablet be dipped in water, preferably warm, before insertion.

(*b*) Some of the foam tablets must be inserted a definite time (three to five minutes) before coitus, to allow the optimum foam production to coincide, as far as possible, with ejaculation. Such accurate timing of coitus has psychological and physical drawbacks.

(*c*) The tablets are stable only in the absence of moisture, and must be kept in an airtight container.

(*d*) The foam may cause sharp pain when there are abrasions. The tablets should not, therefore, be used at the consummation of marriage, or until any consequent abrasions and lacerations of the hymen and vagina have healed. In some cases, too, the foam causes smarting, even in the absence of abrasions.

(*e*) Most foam tablets contain a certain amount of insoluble matter which remains within the vagina unless a douche is used subsequently.

Proprietary foam tablets on the market include the following:—

Agressit (chloramine and cupreine derivatives and an aluminium salt in a foaming base).

Antibion (quinine, boric acid, lactic acid, and formates, in a foaming base).

Antipart (paratoluene sodium sulpho-chloramide, acids glutamic, boric, amido-iso-capronic, tartaric, amido-acetic and adipic, amylum maranthæ, saponin and sodium bicarbonate).

Note.—The foaming solution contains hypochlorous acid, chlorine and oxygen, which are deodorant and disinfectant.

Bircon (chinosol, zinc sulpho-carbolate, starch, sodium bicarbonate and tartaric acid).

Bymeston tablets (perborate of sodium, magnesium silicate, sodium carbonate, citric acid, starch).

Finil (dioxyquinolin sulphate, boric acid, burnt alum, starch, egg albumen, sodium bicarbonate and tartaric acid).

Lomolo (oxyquinoline sulphate and zinc sulphocarbolate, in an effervescing base).

Proseldis foaming tablets (chinosol, boric acid, acid potassium tartrate and sodium bicarbonate).

Semori (ortho-hydroxy-pyridine sulphate, potassium boricotartaric, corpus spumans).

Note.—Corpus spumans contains, among other ingredients, the acid and alkali which form the foam body. The exact composition is not disclosed.

Speton (sodium-dichloro-p-sulphamido benzoate dioxy-succinic acid, lactose, starch and French chalk, sodium bicarbonate and tartaric acid).

Foam Powder (Femfoam).—Dr. De Vilbis, Director of the Mothers' Health Clinics of Florida, is experimenting with a foam powder to be used with a non-fitted rubber sponge pessary. The powder has a base of sulphonated alcohol. She recommends the method for indigent families who are unable to visit a doctor or a clinic.

Preliminary tests of the effects of Femfoam on the vaginal mucous membrane of bitches, conducted by Dr. H. M. Carleton on behalf of the Medical Committee of the National Birth Control Association, London, have not given satisfactory results. Dr. Carleton suggests that the harmful effects observed in his experiments were possibly due to the generation of formaldehyde (September, 1936). The constituents of the foam powder will doubtless be changed to avoid harmful effects.

Comparative Spermicidal Power of Certain Chemical Contraceptives

Unpublished results by Dr. John R. Baker and Mr. R. M. Ransom, communicated to the Medical Sub-Committee of the National Birth Control Association. Printed by kind permission of Dr. Baker (May, 1936).

Note.—Results of tests of total spermicidal power, and not of rate of diffusion, are given.

EXPLANATION OF SYMBOLS

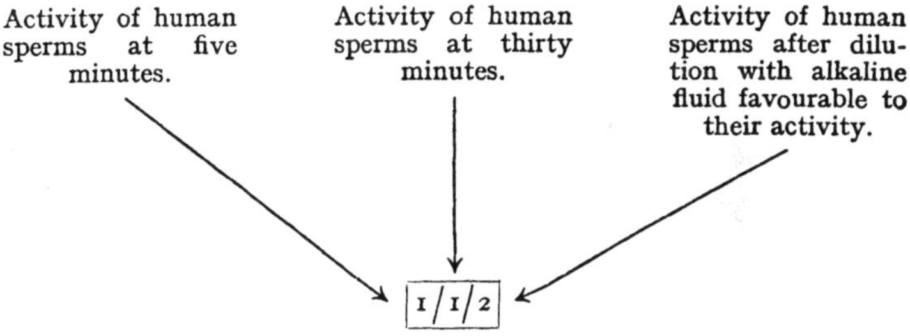

S =	1 suppository, or	2 gm. of	"ointment"	or	"jelly"	to	6	c.c.	of fluid.
$\frac{S}{2}$ =	,,	,,	,,	,,	,,	,,	12	,,	,,
$\frac{S}{4}$ =	,,	,,	,,	,,	,,	,,	24	,,	,,
$\frac{S}{8}$ =	,,	,,	,,	,,	,,	,,	48	,,	,,
$\frac{S}{16}$ =	,,	,,	,,	,,	,,	,,	96	,,	,,
$\frac{S}{32}$ =	,,	,,	,,	,,	,,	,,	192	,,	,,
$\frac{S}{64}$ =	,,	,,	,,	,,	,,	,,	384	,,	,,

	S	$\frac{S}{2}$	$\frac{S}{4}$	$\frac{S}{8}$	$\frac{S}{16}$	$\frac{S}{32}$	$\frac{S}{64}$
M.3.A. .		0/0/0	0/0/0	0/0/0	0/0/0, 3/0/0	3/3/—	1/1/1
Semori[1] .	0/0/0	0/0/1					
Prensol .	0/0/0, 0/0/0, 0/0/0	1+/1/2	2+/2+/2+				
Rendell's "Wife's Friend."	0/0/0, 0/0/0, 1/0/0	1/1/1	1/0/0	2+/2/3			
Prentifs .	0/0/1, 0/0/0	3/3/—					
Bircon .	0/0/0, 1/1/0	2/1/1	2/2/0				
Mil-San .	0/0/1, 0/0/2, 0/0/2+	0/0/2	1/1/1				
Orthogynol	2+/1+/1, 3/3/3						
G.P. soluble	3/3/—, 2+/2+/3, 2+/2+/—						
G.P. ointment.	3/3/—, 3/3/—	3/3/3					
G.P. jelly .	3/3/—, 3/3/—						

[1] Tests not completed.

Effects of Chemicals on the Vagina and Uterus

The importance of adequate experimental tests on animals of the harmlessness of chemical contraceptives, before clinical application, cannot be over-estimated. The average latent period in the production of an irritation carcinoma is estimated to be about twelve years; and Dr. H. M. Carleton ("Chemical Control of Conception") expresses the view that naked eye detection of minute and incipient vaginal and cervical lesions is unlikely in the examination of the vagina and cervix with a speculum.

Only substances which have been proved experimentally to be non-irritating to the vaginal and uterine mucosæ should be prescribed for clinical use.

At the suggestion of the Birth Control Investigation Committee, experiments have been conducted by Drs. H. M. Carleton and H. W. Florey to determine some effects of common contraceptives on the vaginal and uterine mucosæ.

The following is an extract from their published report

(*The Journal of Obstetrics and Gynæcology of the British Empire,* " Birth Control Studies," Vol. 38, No. 3).

Summary

" 1. Repeated daily injections have been made *per vaginum* in rabbits, cats and dogs.

" 2. The following substances were tested:

antibion,
chinosol (in cocoa-butter),
finil,
quinine (double strength in cocoa-butter and gelatine),
semori,
speton,
spetonex,
quinine and urea.

" 3. Of these, antibion, chinosol, quinine (in cocoa-butter and gelatine), semori and speton, did not produce any observable lesions of the vaginal mucosa. Some shedding of the mucosa was noted subsequently to the injection of finil, but there was not any inflammation. Possibly the desquamation did not exceed physiological limits.

" 4. Spetonex caused ulceration of the vaginal mucous membrane in rabbits, but did not have any effect on that of dogs.

" 5. Quinine and urea regularly produced an intense vaginitis in both rabbits and dogs.

" 6. The uterine horn was directly injected in rabbits with the following substances: chinosol, very dilute formalin, quinine, semori, quinine and urea.

" 7. Chinosol, quinine (double strength in cocoa-butter) and semori were found not to have any effect on the normal endometrium of rabbits.

" 8. Formol was likewise harmless in concentrations up to just under $\frac{1}{8}$ per cent.

" 9. Quinine and urea in certain concentrations produced necrosis and sloughing of the endometrium."

PermFoam.—Dr. Carleton found PermFoam to be harmless to the vagina of bitches (" Chemical Control of Conception," 1933, chapter on Pathology of Contraception).

Prensols.—Half a " Prensol " suppository was placed in the vagina of a bitch daily for a fortnight (except Sundays). Dr. Carleton reported on the sectioned vagina as follows : " No microscopic evidence of damage. Occasional leucocytes in the mucosa : probably, however, these are within physiological limits."

It should be noted that it was impossible to reproduce exactly the routine contraceptive procedure of many women, who use chemical contraceptives at varying intervals over periods of several years. In these experiments, daily injections and relatively large doses were used.

Moreover, only bitches have a stratified squamous vaginal epithelium similar to that of women. The vaginal epithelium of the rabbit is more delicate and the upper portion has a columnar epithelium ; and in cats the upper vaginal mucous membrane is transitional in type. In the case of the rabbits used in these experiments, however, a control experiment was conducted, in which a catheter was passed for twenty-seven consecutive days ; there was no evidence of trauma.

The possibility of the aspiration or the injection of chemicals from the vagina into the uterus cannot yet be ruled out, although up to the present experiments conducted on animals to determine this point have had negative results.

Possibility of Genetic Modification of Sperms by Chemical Contraceptives

It is important to exclude definitely the possibility of injury to the sperm without the destruction of its fertilising power by a sub-lethal dose of a chemical spermicide. A sperm with damaged nuclear constituents may produce harmful recessive mutations. With this investigation in view, a scheme has been drawn up by Professor J. B. S. Haldane, at the request of the Birth Control Investigation Committee, for an experiment involving the inbreeding, on a large scale, of the F_1 generation of rabbits. This investigation is to be made when the most suitable combination of chemical and vehicle has been found.

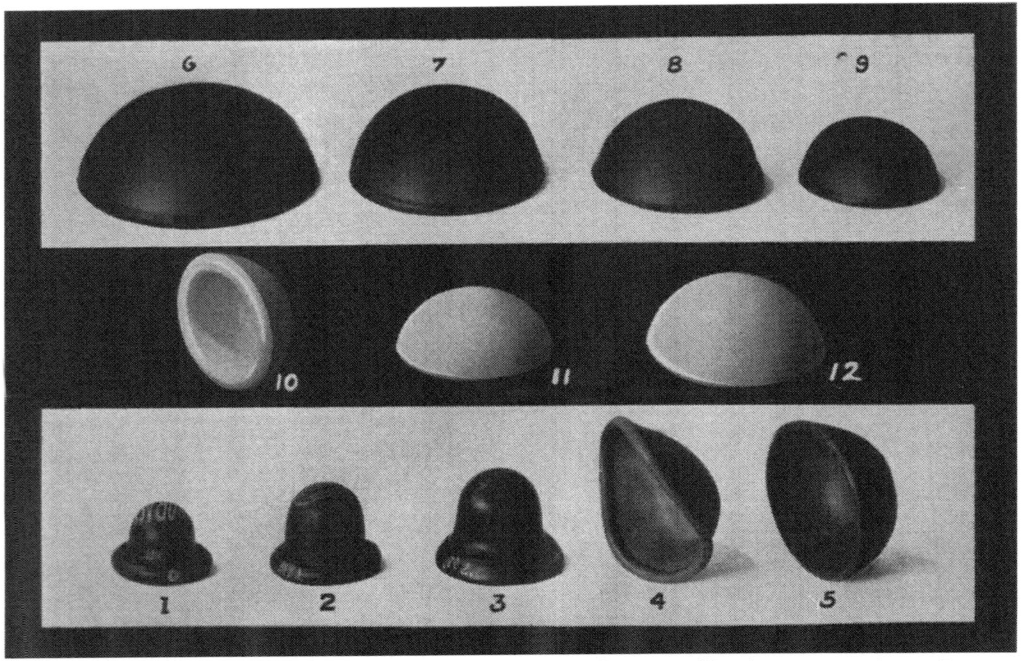

1. Prorace. 2. Racial. 3. Unique. 4. Matrisalus. 5. Dutch or Mensinga. 6, 7, 8, 9. Four Dutch Pessaries (to show variation in size). 10, 11, 12. Dumas (small, medium and large size).

[To face p. 65.

CHAPTER IV

METHODS OF CONTRACEPTION

OCCLUSIVE PESSARIES

Occlusive Pessaries.—The occlusive pessaries, like the sheath, prevent contact between the ejaculate and the cervix; but, unlike the sheath, they permit the semen to be deposited in the vagina. OCCLUSIVE PESSARIES, THEREFORE, SHOULD BE USED ONLY IN CONJUNCTION WITH ONE OR MORE CHEMICAL SPERMICIDES (*e.g.*, spermicidal lubricant and subsequent medicated douching, or spermicidal lubricant and a chemical contraceptive (jelly, suppository or foam tablet), since the sperms must be prevented from ascending into the uterus after the removal of the pessary.

Classification.—Unnecessary confusion has arisen owing to differences in the classification of occlusive pessaries. They are herein classified thus:—

A. Cervical "caps."
B. Vault pessaries.
C. Diaphragms.

General Considerations.—The occlusive pessary has the great advantage of permitting the spontaneity and normal sequence of coitus, since it can be adjusted before retiring, and may be left in position until the following morning.

So that the use of an occlusive pessary shall not be actually or potentially harmful, the following conditions should be fulfilled:—

(*a*) There should be no constriction of the cervix.

(*b*) There should be free drainage for the cervical secretion.

(*c*) The removal of the pessary should not involve a pull upon the uterus.

It is at least possible that the rim of a cervical pessary, which exerts only moderate pressure (sufficient to prevent it from slipping off a moist, conical cervix) when it is first adjusted, may become a harmfully constricting band during the vascular changes which occur during sexual excitement. During detumescence there should be no obstruction to the vascular changes involved in a return to the normal.

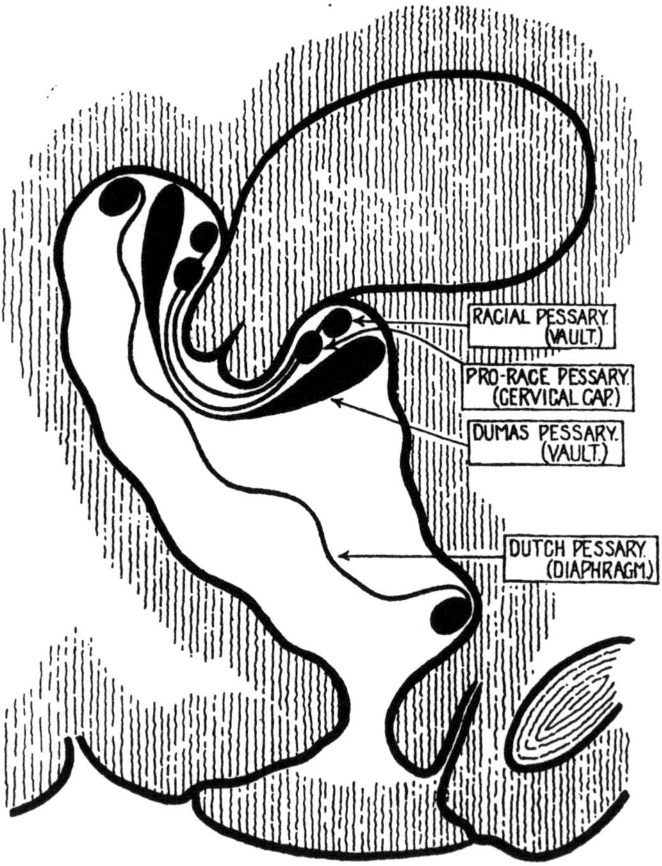

DIAGRAM ILLUSTRATING FORMS OF OCCLUSIVE PESSARY

The orthodox anatomy book picture of the female genital tract gives the impression of a cervix practically in contact with the vaginal walls, so that a cervical cap would derive some support from the surrounding vagina until the vaginal cavity was distended during coitus.

In my experience, especially among clinic patients, this condition is rarely met with. In the large roomy vagina of the woman who has borne children the cervix protrudes into a relatively large cavity, and a cervical pessary in such a case must depend upon suction, and upon the grip of its rim on the cervix, in order to maintain its position. It must be noted that in many cases the vaginal cervix is conical in shape, and the lubricated pessary would tend to slip off the moist mucous membrane.

Dr. Helena Wright reports three cases of women who had used a cervical cap three or four times a week, in which "slight abrasions of the mucous membrane were found round the outer edges of the lower face of the cervix," which "healed rapidly when the use of the cap was suspended" ("Practice of Contraception," Sanger and Stone, p. 16).

There are obvious disadvantages in wearing, for some hours, a cap which holds up the secretions in contact with the cervix, as do the small portio caps and the pro-race type with the low dome. One has no guarantee that patients will faithfully observe the rule as to the maximum time an occlusive pessary may remain in position without probable injurious effects.

Dr. Hans Hehfeldt, of Berlin, in a paper[1] read at the Seventh International Birth Control Conference, Zurich, 1930, remarks:—

> "A cap that fits tightly over the cervix impedes the secretions, and any action of this kind causes inflammation of tissues when there is such tendency. Although this action upon the secretion only lasts a few hours, it must not be forgotten that it is recurrent and takes place every time the pessary is used. The effect can be cumulative and cause a return of an old inflammation, as we have frequently been able to observe."

The cumulative effect of the repeated drag upon the cervix which is involved in the removal of certain types of pessaries which fit closely on to the cervix may cause

[1] "The Physical and Psychological Aspects of Birth Control in the Light of Experience in Private Practice and in Birth Control Clinics."

such stretching and weakening of the uterine supports as to lead to prolapsus uteri.

The writer was, in one case, at a loss to account for a marked prolapse of the uterus in a well-to-do healthy patient of thirty-seven, who had a history of two normal confinements twelve and fifteen years ago respectively. For the past eight years she had used, two or three times a week, a cervical pessary, which she produced for inspection.

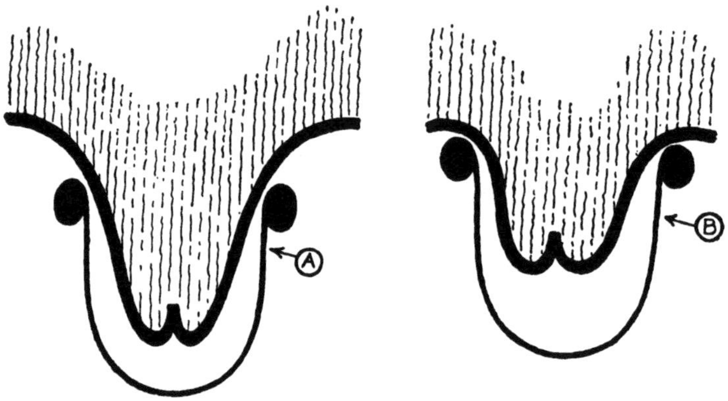

EXAMPLE OF THE USE OF THE SAME PESSARY IN TWO WAYS

A. Occlusive pessary used as a CERVICAL CAP on a long conical cervix. (I consider this fitting to be potentially harmful because of the possible constriction of the cervix by the rim of the pessary, and of the inadequate space for the normal cervical secretions.

B. The same appliance used as a VAULT PESSARY over a short cervix. (This fitting is probably harmless provided the usual conditions for the use of an occlusive pessary are observed.)

It was impossible to remove this pessary without pronounced pull on the cervix, and she herself had noted this fact. The conclusion was that the prolapse was probably due to the use of this type of pessary. Subsequent clinical experience has supported this conclusion.

Wright, in the paper from which the previous extract is taken, states that "In two patients who had normally anteverted uterine fundi, a pronounced retroversion was produced after some months of the use of this cap."

Choice of Type of Pessary.—Each patient presents an

individual problem which cannot be settled without a pelvic examination. The choice of an occlusive pessary is determined primarily by the anatomical pelvic condition—the shape and size of the vagina, the tone of the peri-vaginal muscles and the presence of scarring, adhesions or other vaginal abnormalities, the position and condition of the cervix and uterine fundus.

The writer regards the diaphragm pessary, fitted in the oblique position in suitable cases, as the most satisfactory type of pessary in regard to reliability, ease of adjustment and removal, and harmlessness. Whether the diaphragm pessary is suitable in any particular case depends upon the factors stated above. The routine use of the diaphragm pessary, irrespective of the anatomical conditions, must lead to discomfort and other unsatisfactory results in certain cases. The remedy in such cases is to substitute a different type of pessary or other mechanical contraceptive.

The indications and contra-indications for the use of the various types of occlusive pessaries are discussed under the appropriate headings.

Cervical Pessaries.—In my classification cervical caps include all those which fit on to the vaginal cervix, *and do not depend upon contact with the vault of the vagina for support.* These caps include :—

(*a*) "PORTIO" CAPS.—These are cup-like pessaries which fit closely on to the vaginal cervix, and do not come into contact with the vaginal vault. They are made in hard metal (gold, silver, aluminium, etc.), soft pliable metal, and celluloid. They maintain their position by close fit and by suction.

They have the following disadvantages :—

1. Constriction of the cervix, interfering with vascular changes.

2. Damming back of the secretions. Some modified forms have valves, etc., which are claimed to permit free drainage of the uterine secretions.

3. Drag on the uterus during removal.

Portio caps are little used in this country. I consider them to be harmful.

(*b*) SHALLOW-DOMED RUBBER CERVICAL CAPS, with a solid or hollow flexible rim.

This type of pessary, which includes the Pro-race and similar forms, is popular with many doctors. Being flexible, and having a deeper dome that the " portio " caps, it is less potentially harmful; but I consider its use as a *cervical* cap unjustifiable for reasons given under " General Considerations." It is definitely contra-indicated in any pathological condition of the cervix such as cervical erosion, ulceration or laceration. Leucorrhœa, from whatever cause, is also a contra-indication to its use.

(*c*) DEEP-DOMED CERVICAL CAPS of a size not large enough to allow contact between the rim of the cap and the vaginal vault.

These caps are usually made in four sizes: 0, 1, 2, 3.

There are many variations of the cervical cap. Modifications include air-inflated rims, solid hard rims, rims of rubber covered spiral springs, special contrivances to permit escape of secretions, sponge covered domes, etc.

> *Note.*—The writer classifies " cervical caps " of a size large enough to permit contact of rim with vaginal vault as *vault* pessaries. When such large caps are used in this way, constriction of the cervix can be avoided.

Vault Pessaries.—This group includes all those which maintain their position by contact with the vaginal vault; they may or may not be supported externally by the vaginal wall, according to the tone of the vaginal muscles and the size of the cavity of the upper vagina. Unlike the diaphragm pessary, they do not cover any part of the vaginal walls.

Types used as vault pessaries include:—

(*a*) THE RACIAL, a modification of the Pro-race designed by Dr. Marie Stopes and approved by the Medical Committee of the Constructive Birth Control Society. It has a solid flexible rubber rim and a deep dome of thin rubber, and is made in four sizes: 0, 1, 2, 3.

(*b*) THE " CERCAP," the same shape as the " Racial," but made by the moulding process.

(*c*) THE " GAMOPHILE " Cervical Cap, prepared according

to directions of Van de Velde, with deep latex rubber dome of condom thinness and soft rubber rim.

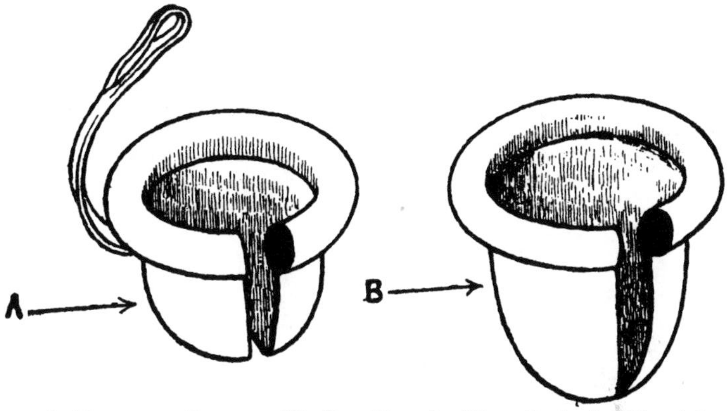

A. Pro-race Pessary (Shallow Dome). The attached rubber tab is to facilitate the removal of the pessary.
B. Racial Pessary (Deep Dome). This may be used as a cervical cap or as a vault pessary, according to the relative size and shape of the cervix.

(*d*) The Unique Pessary has a solid rubber rim and thin deep rubber dome.

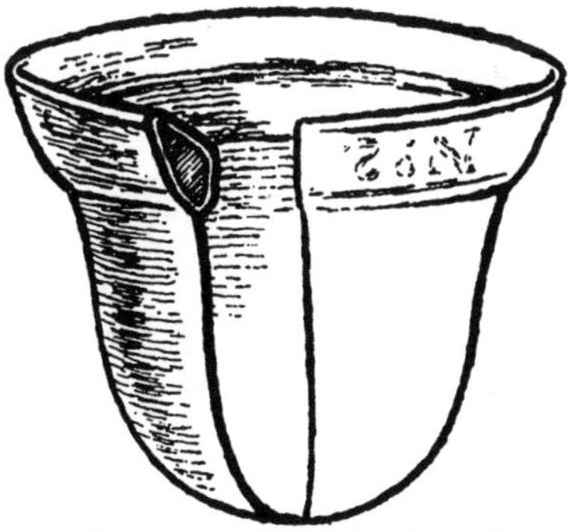

Unique Pessary. Section removed to show shape of the solid rubber rim.

(*e*) The Dumas or French Pessary.—The original form ("Antigeniture"), made of thick, hard rubber, was very shallow and shaped somewhat like a watchglass. It was suitable only for cases of very short vaginal cervix and of amputated cervix. On a normal cervix such a cap would not be in contact with the vaginal vault ; it would, therefore,

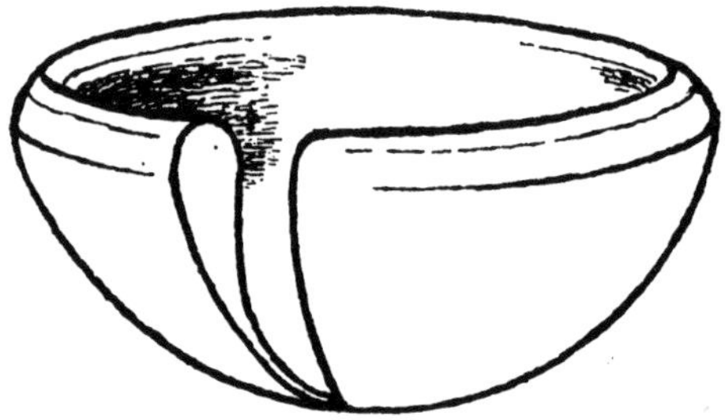

DUMAS PESSARY. Section removed to show varying thickness of the rubber dome and the solid rubber rim.

fail to occlude completely the cervix, and would readily tilt during coitus.

The modifications now in use at British Birth Control Clinics are a great improvement on the original form ; they are made of softer rubber, and have deeper domes. There are three sizes—small, medium and large. However, their usefulness continues to be limited by the depth of the dome, which is still too shallow for the long vaginal cervix.

Dumas pessaries include :—

Prencap Dumas-type pessary, with thin rubber dome and solid grooved rubber rim. The object of the grooved rim

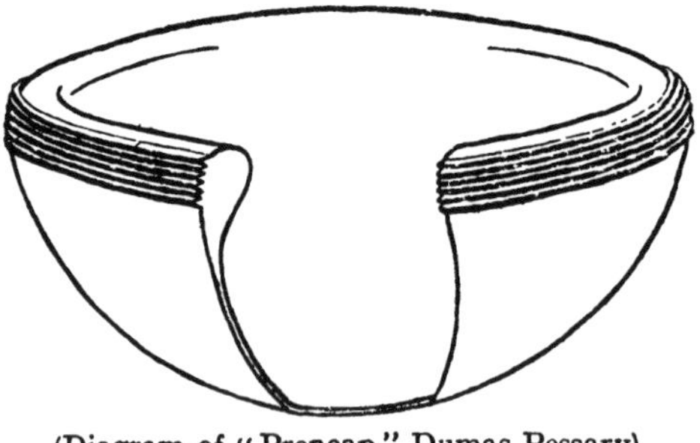

(Diagram of "Prencap" Dumas Pessary).

is to retain the spermicidal jelly in contact with the vaginal vault. The writer has found these caps particularly useful in cases of excessive vaginal secretions, as the grooved rim appears to check the tendency of the pessary to slip down in the excessively lubricated vagina.

The Dumas is *unsuitable* :—

1. Where a *long* cervix prevents the rim from fitting up closely against the vaginal vault.
2. Where the pessary is likely to be dislodged by the phallus during coitus. This tends to happen when the position of the uterus is normal, so that the cervical axis is roughly at right angles to the vaginal axis.
3. In cases of leucorrhœa. The secretions would collect in the shallow dome, in contact with cervical tissue.
4. Where the relative shortness of the patient's fingers renders difficult or impossible the adjustment and removal of the pessary.

(*f*) SMALL-SIZED DUTCH (MENSINGA) OR RAMSES DIAPHRAGM, used in the alternative vault position (see p. 86). It then acts as a vault pessary, as the anterior rim is

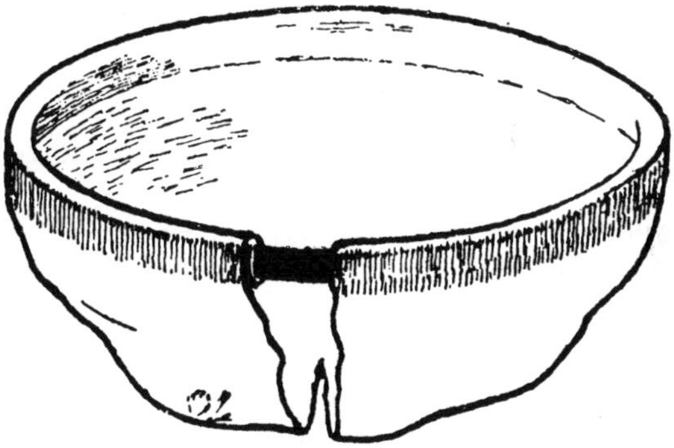

DUTCH OR MENSINGA PESSARY. Section removed to show watch-spring in rim.

pushed up into the anterior fornix, leaving the anterior wall of the vagina exposed.

Where there are pathological secretions, it is desirable that any vault pessary should be used only during coitus and not left in the vagina for some hours.

Note.—Cervical and vault pessaries are easier to adjust

and less likely to be dislodged during coitus, when the uterus is in such a position (retroversion, acute anteflexion) as to bring its axis into line with the vaginal axis.

Diaphragm Pessaries.—These pessaries divide the vagina diagonally into two parts :—

1. An anterior and upper portion, including the cervix, the anterior fornix and the upper part of the vaginal wall.

2. A posterior and lower portion, which admits the phallus in coitus.

Diaphragm pessaries differ in shape, depth of dome, type of rim and kind of rubber. They include :—

(*a*) THE DUTCH (MENSINGA OR HAIRE) PESSARY has a circular, rubber-covered watch-spring rim, enclosing a thin rubber dome. It has been used extensively in Holland since 1885, where it was popularised by Dr. Mensinga.

(*b*) THE RAMSES has a coiled wire spring in place of the watch-spring of the Dutch pessary, and the rim is therefore more pliable. The deeper dome permits part of the diaphragm to be rolled round the rim.

The " Lam-butt " cap with " Duplex Rim " is a diaphragm pessary with an outer spiral spring covering an inner watch spring.

The Gamophile diaphragm, prepared according to directions of Van de Velde, has a spiral spring rim and a dome of latex rubber of condom thinness.

The Holland-Rantos " Koromex " diaphragm has a rubber covered coil spring rim and a thin rubber dome.

> *Note.*—The coil spring rims are especially suitable for the hypersensitive vagina.

(*c*) THE MATRISALUS is adapted for patients with cystocele, prolapse, lacerations of the perinæum and relaxed vaginal walls. The shape of the rim resembles that of a Hodge or Smith pessary, and the pessary is used so that the crossbar rests behind the symphisis, and extra support is given to the lower part of the anterior vaginal wall.

The Holland-Rantos Matrisalus diaphragm (coil spring rim) is made in sizes 1, 2, 3, 4 and 5.

(*d*) THE GAMOPHILE RETROFLEXION HODGE-SMITH MODEL, prepared according to directions of Van de Velde, has a spiral spring shaped like a Hodge-Smith pessary and a latex rubber dome of condom thinness. The dome has its most pronounced curvature upwards and to the front so that it adapts itself to the position of the cervix in acute retroflexion of the uterus. It is supplied in sizes from 60 mm. to 100 mm. (long axis) by steps of 5 mm.

Fittings and Sizes.—The sizes of the circular diaphragm pessaries are the measurements in millimetres of their diameters. The usual range of sizes of diaphragm pessaries extends from 45 mm. to 90 mm., in steps of 2½ mm. Gamophile diaphragms are made in sizes ranging from 50 mm. to 80 mm., in steps of 5 mm. Holland-Rantos "Koromex" diaphragms are made in sizes ranging from 50 mm. to 105 mm., in steps of 5 mm.

Fitting-rims, without the diaphragms, are available for determining the correct size for the patient. The general practitioner whose birth control practice is not sufficiently large to justify the expense of stocking a complete set of pessaries could use the fitting rings for determining the correct size for a patient at the first consultation; and instruction in the use of the pessary could be deferred until a subsequent visit, when her pessary is available.

Since rubber tends to perish, it is unwise to keep stocks of pessaries for more than a few months.

The correct size of pessary can be determined only by gynæcological examination and actual trial of the pessary or fitting-rim; it is impossible to judge the size in any other way. There is no relation between the size of the pessary required and the number of children borne by the patient. A size which is correct when fitted a month or so after marriage may be too small within six months; and a pessary fitted shortly after confinement may be too large when the tissues have regained their tone. A nervous patient, on her first visit for a fitting, may not succeed in relaxing sufficiently for the final fitting to be made; she may need the substitution of a pessary one or two sizes larger on her return visit in a week's time. The doctor should arrange for re-examinations at intervals of three to six months.

Advantages of the Diaphragm Pessaries

1. There is no pressure or constriction of the cervical tissues.

2. There is no interference with the physiological vascular changes of the cervix during coitus.

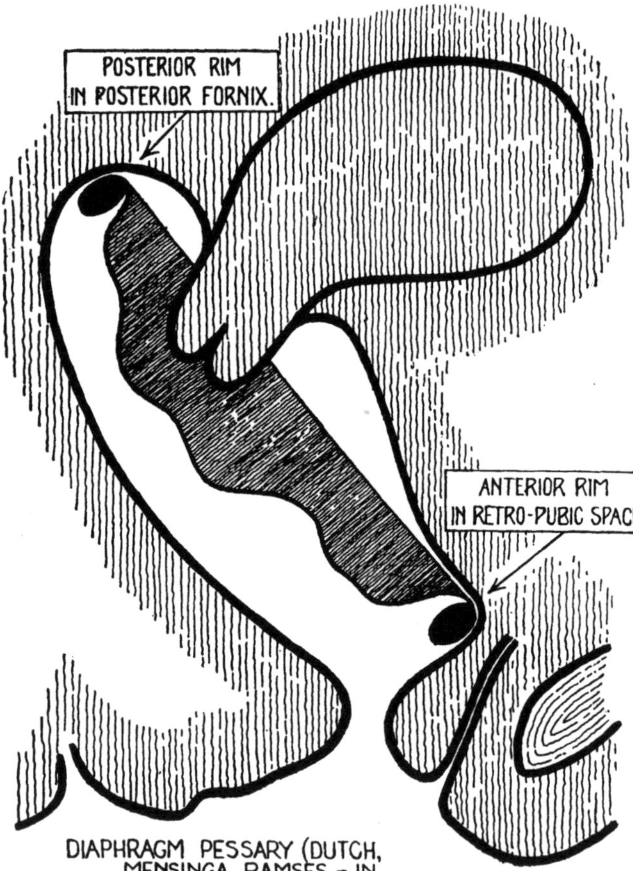

DIAPHRAGM PESSARY (DUTCH, MENSINGA, RAMSES – IN USUAL OBLIQUE FITTING.)

3. Secretions can flow away freely into the loose-fitting diaphragm out of contact with the cervix.

4. The position of the uterus is generally immaterial provided that the rim can obtain adequate support from

the vaginal walls, and provided that the patient can be successfully instructed to adjust the pessary.

5. A lacerated cervix, which is commonly found after childbirth, is not a contra-indication to its use.

6. It is easy to adjust and remove.

Disadvantages of the Diaphragm Pessaries

1. The rim of the pessary may hamper the physiological contractions of the perivaginal muscles in coitus. *The Gamophile retroflexion Hodge-Smith model diaphragm pessary is claimed to avoid any impediment to the action of the vaginal muscles. The amount of interference with muscular contractions will depend largely upon the tension of the rim of the pessary. The rim should be as flexible as is compatible with its maintaining uniform contact with the vaginal walls. The rims of some makes of diaphragm pessaries are much too stiff.*

2. A loaded rectum, by causing irregular bulging of the posterior vaginal wall, may prevent the satisfactory occlusion of the cervix. In the usual coital attitude, with the woman in the dorsal position, the seminal pool collects in the posterior fornix ; and semen may possibly ooze past the rim of the pessary through a space caused by the pressure of fæcal masses in the rectum.

3. If there be beneficial absorption of semen from the whole of the vaginal surface, as is maintained by Stopes and others, then it may be a disadvantage that a relatively large area of vaginal mucous membrane should be cut off from contact with the seminal fluid. The probability is, however, that sufficient absorption could take place through the exposed posterior vaginal wall.

As is the case with any other type of occlusive pessary, the diaphragm pessary must be used properly if it is to give satisfactory results ; it must be of the correct size and correctly adjusted, and it must not be used by patients for whom it is unsuitable. We have ample clinical evidence that, in suitable cases, neither partner is conscious of the presence of the pessary during coitus, nor of any lessening of sexual satisfaction.

Diaphragm Pessary used in the Original "Oblique"

Position.—The diaphragm pessary is inserted into a position similar to that of a ring pessary used in the treatment of prolapsus uteri. The rim rests posteriorly in the posterior fornix and anteriorly in the depression behind the pubic bone; it therefore encloses the portio, the vaginal vault, and also the anterior wall of the vagina. The support given by the pubic bone anteriorly, when the pessary is correctly fitted, prevents it from slipping down and protruding from the vulva when the patient coughs or strains. The rim should fit uniformly, *as closely to the vaginal surface as is consistent with the avoidance of harmful or uncomfortable pressure:* and the patient should not be conscious of its presence in the vagina. I advise inserting the pessary convex side towards the cervix for two reasons:—

1. The gutter formed between rim and diaphragm impedes the oozing of the semen between the rim of the pessary and the vaginal mucous membrane.
2. It is much easier to remove the pessary by hooking the finger tip into this gutter than by forcing the finger over the rim.

The physical conditions which are essential for the proper use of the diaphragm pessary are that there should be:—

1. A retro-pubic space which permits the anterior part of the rim of the pessary to be supported adequately by the pubic bone.

   If this space is absent or inadequate the rim of the pessary slips down in front when the patient coughs or strains, or even without increase of intra-abdominal pressure. Such projection of the rim anteriorly would cause discomfort during coitus; and the pessary might slip down sufficiently to expose the cervix.

   The retro-pubic space is obliterated in cases of cystocele; it is absent also in certain cases in which the pelvic condition is healthy.

2. Sufficient tone in the vaginal and perineal muscles to hold the pessary in position.

   It cannot be used, therefore, in those cases where the vaginal walls and perineal muscles have been badly damaged through childbirth or from other causes, especially where a badly torn perineum has not been successfully repaired.

3. Absence of adhesions or other abnormalities which distort the vaginal canal.

A distended rectum will cause the use of a diaphragm pessary to be uncomfortable and unreliable. The constipation should be corrected before the patient is allowed to use a diaphragm pessary.

In my opinion, so long as there is adequate support for the rim of the pessary, the actual position of the cervix is of no great importance, provided that the patient can be taught to adjust the pessary correctly.

Konikow states that acute anteversion and retroversion are contra-indications to the use of the diaphragm pessary, but I have patients with these uterine displacements who are using the diaphragm pessary with complete comfort and success.

Obviously, if a retroversion were associated with a greatly enlarged fundus which partially obliterated the posterior fornix, then there would be interference with the fit of a diaphragm pessary ; and a retroverted tender fundus would cause discomfort from contact with the rim of the pessary. The large majority of such cases would, in my opinion, be unsuitable for any occlusive device.

The Technique.—The pessary, lubricated with a spermicidal ointment or jelly, can be inserted as early as two or three hours before coitus if necessary, but *it should not remain in the vagina for longer than about twelve hours*, and it should be worn for as short a time as possible in cases of leucorrhœa when the discharge is profuse.

The disadvantage of inserting the pessary some considerable time before it is needed is that, owing to the lateral pressure of the vaginal walls (perivaginal muscles) during the movements of walking, standing, etc., the rim of the pessary becomes bent into a pronounced oval outline ; during coitus in the position with the thighs everted, the lateral fit of the distorted pessary may be so defective as to lessen its effectiveness. For maximum security I advise the patient to insert the pessary when she retires, so that it may retain more closely its circular shape during coitus.

If, however, the pessary has been inserted some considerable time before coitus, it is desirable that the patient should, shortly before coitus, confirm the correctness of the position of the pessary.

Need for Further Measures (suppository, tablet, jelly or douche).—Since the longevity of sperms in the vagina is not conclusively determined, and is certainly variable, the pessary should not be removed until steps have been taken to destroy those sperms which are present in the ejaculate within the vagina. Some may have been killed or immobilised by the spermicidal lubricant on the rubber pessary, but many thousands of sperms, each one of them capable of ascending into the uterus and fertilising the ovum, may be held up in the folds and pockets of the vaginal mucous membrane, even though most of the semen has flowed out of the vagina.

Two possible methods of dealing with the living spermatozoa in the vagina are :—

1. Spermicidal jelly, ointment, suppository or tablet may be inserted, after the pessary is in place, but *before* coitus.
2. A medicated or plain water douche may be used before removing the pessary, and again immediately after ; that is to say, the removal of the pessary should take place midway in the douching process.

Considering the nature of the vaginal cavity, the effectiveness of the spermicidal preparation used depends not only upon its spermicidal power, but also upon its surface tension and distribution. The foaming preparations and the douche administered with sufficient pressure to distend the vagina and thus open up the folds and furrows of the vaginal mucous membrane are probably more widely distributed than the cocoa-butter and gelatine suppositories, although one must remember that the movements of the phallus during coitus assist the distribution of both foaming and non-foaming preparations.

In addition to the spermicidal lubricant on the rim and diaphragm of the pessary, a second line of defence should be provided by the insertion into the upper vagina of a

PLATE I

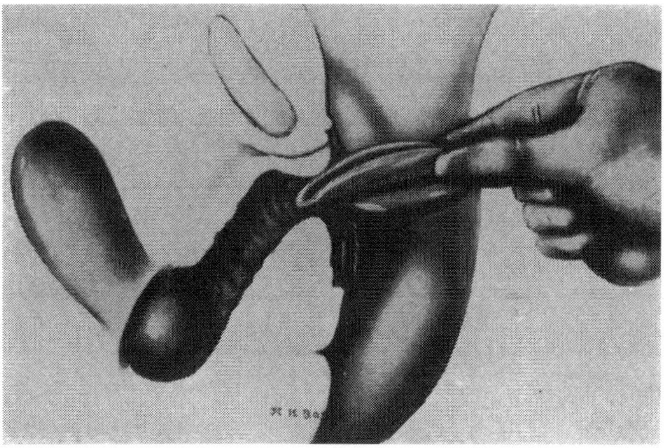

Adjustment of Diaphragm Pessary

First Stage

The pessary is held compressed between the thumb and finger, the convex side towards the abdomen.

If the direction here shown were continued within the vagina, the entering posterior part of the rim would slide into the anterior fornix instead of passing below the cervix into the posterior fornix. To avoid the projecting cervix, when a portion of the pessary has entered the vagina, the direction in which the pessary is pushed to complete the insertion must be altered to direct the rim behind the cervix into the posterior fornix.

(*Reproduced by permission of Dr. Hannah Stone.*)

[*To face p.* 80.

PLATE II

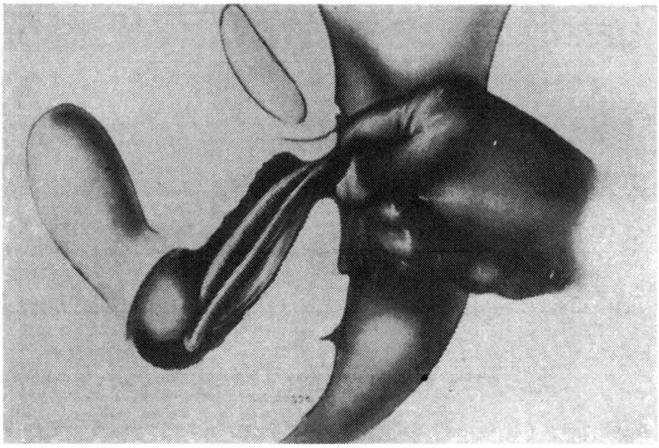

Second Stage

The pessary is pushed along the posterior vaginal wall past the cervix. Where the cervix is especially prominent, it is helpful to direct the posterior rim with the index finger between the pessary and the posterior vaginal wall, the finger tip in the groove between the rim and the rubber diaphragm. In this way the rim can be hooked round the projecting cervix. The Janvier thumb method is an alternative procedure. (See Plate V.)

(*Reproduced by permission of Dr. Hannah Stone.*)

PLATE III

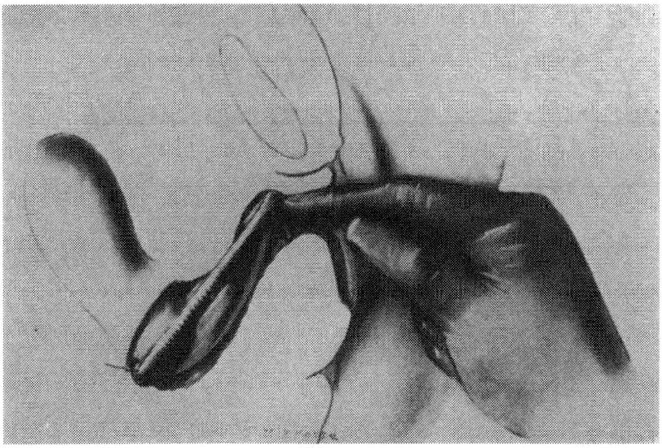

Third Stage

The pessary is now correctly placed, the insertion being completed by the index finger pushing the anterior rim into the retro-pubic space. The cervix, the vaginal vault and the anterior vaginal wall are enclosed by the rubber diaphragm.

(Reproduced by permission of Dr. Hannah Stone.)

PLATE IV

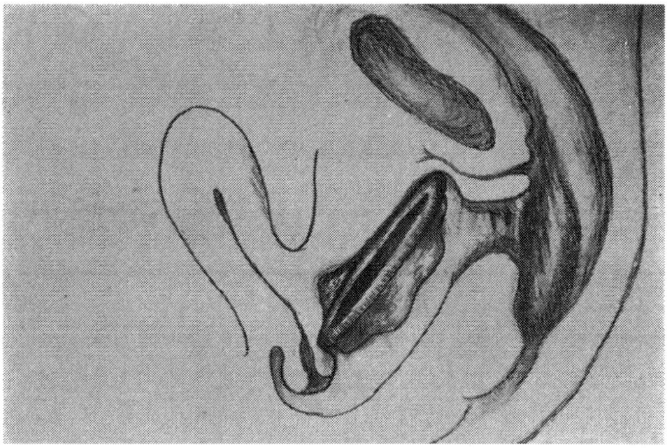

DIAPHRAGM PESSARY INCORRECTLY PLACED

The cervix has been pushed aside, and is exposed in the posterior fornix.

Note. In the large oblique fitting which I advocate, where the pessary rim reaches from the posterior fornix to the retro-pubic space, a pessary placed as here illustrated would protrude anteriorly at the vulva or would compress the cervix and unduly stretch the vaginal wall. It would therefore be uncomfortable or definitely painful.

In any case the error should be detected by the routine check of feeling for the cervix through the thin rubber diaphragm.

(*Reproduced by permission of Dr. Hannah Stone.*)

PLATE V

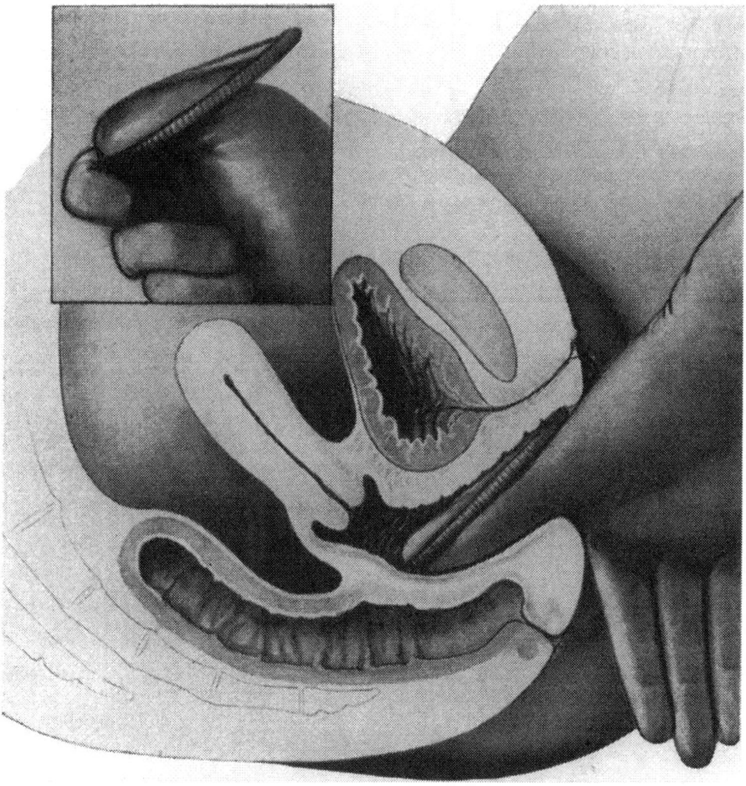

THE JANVIER THUMB METHOD OF INSERTING THE DIAPHRAGM

(Reproduced from the Holland-Rantos "Improved Guide," by permission of Prentif Ltd., London, agents for the Holland-Rantos Co. Inc., New York.)

PLATE VI

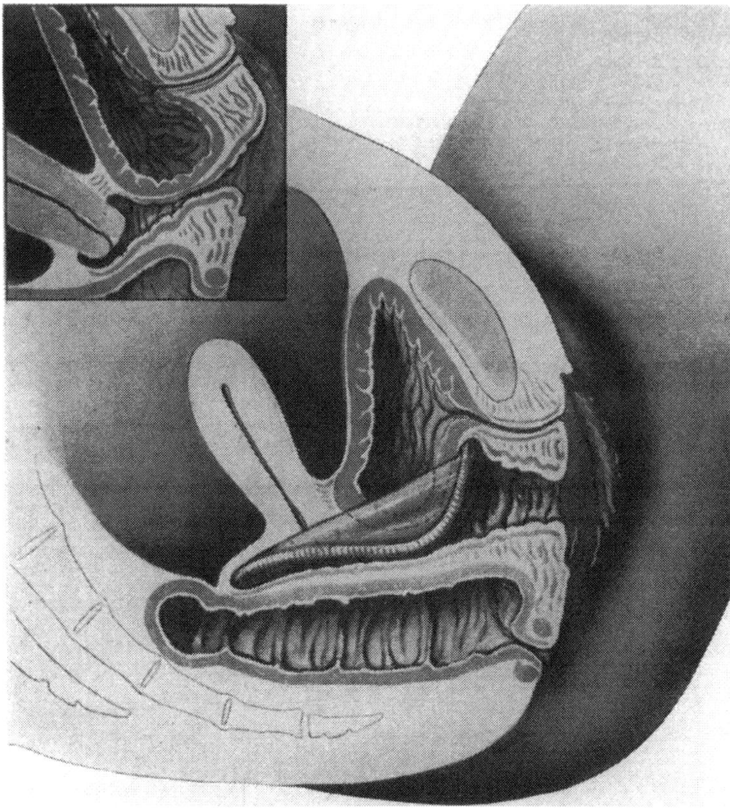

THE H-R MATRISALUS

This is an occlusive diaphragm of special shape, indicated in cases of cystocele or prolapse, where owing to relaxed vaginal walls the ordinary diaphragm cannot be retained in position. It is manufactured in five sizes. The physician should select the largest that can be worn with comfort. The raised part of the rim should fit snugly behind the symphysis.

(Reproduced from the Holland-Rantos "Improved Guide," by permission of Prentif Ltd., London, agents for the Holland-Rantos Co. Inc., New York.)

spermicidal jelly, suppository or tablet before coitus, or by a post-coital douche of plain or medicated water, to wash out the vagina before and after removing the pessary.

I must emphasise that *the occlusive pessary should not be left in the healthy vagina for longer than about twelve hours :* pent up secretions in due course undergo putrefactive changes in the vagina. An interval of several hours between coitus and the subsequent removal of the occlusive pessary is advisable for the following reasons :—

> There is evidence that in some cases the sperms fail to survive many hours within the vagina, even in the absence of spermicides.
>
> It is undesirable to interfere with the normal sequence of coitus by interrupting the post-coital rest and sleep in order to prepare and administer a douche, or to remove and cleanse the pessary.

After the removal of the pessary the circular shape of the rim should be restored by gentle pressure between thumb and finger. The pessary should be washed in soapy water, rinsed with clear water, *thoroughly dried* (with particular attention to the junction of rim and diaphragm), powdered with French chalk or talc powder, and stored in a cool, dry atmosphere, and preferably in the dark. In the tropics the rubber may be smeared with glycerine.

FITTING AND INSTRUCTION OF PATIENT.—*Preparation of Patient.*—Before entering the consulting room the patient should be instructed to empty the bladder (and bowel if necessary) and to wash the hands thoroughly, with special care of the nails.

1. After taking the usual medical history, some time should be given to explaining to the patient, with the help of models or diagrams if available, the object and use of an occlusive pessary.

I recommend giving to the patient a brief and simple outline of the anatomy of the vagina and uterus, so that she may understand clearly the importance of covering the cervix, and so that she may be reassured that there is no danger of a pessary "going too far" and "getting lost inside the body."

2. With the patient in the dorsal or lateral position on the examination couch, a general pelvic examination should be made, and any abnormalities recorded for future reference. Any contra-indications to the use of a pessary would be discovered during this examination, and an alternative method selected if necessary.

3. The correct type and size of pessary should then be determined by trial, and the pessary adjusted.

Experience enables one to estimate the size of a diaphragm pessary with fair accuracy from manual examination of the vagina, but the final test is with the pessary in position. With the diaphragm pessary used in the original oblique method, I use the largest size which is perfectly comfortable to the patient, *and which is not dislodged from the retro-pubic space when the patient coughs and strains.* Almost invariably the patient cannot feel the pessary in the vagina. The rim of the pessary should be in contact with the vaginal surface if possible throughout its circumference, but particularly posteriorly.

4. *Instruction of Patient.*—The utmost patience and thoroughness in teaching the patient are essential, as the success of the method depends upon the correct adjustment of the pessary.

My procedure is as follows :—

(*a*) I instruct the patient, with the pessary in position, to make a digital exploration of the vagina.

The majority of women find the squatting position most convenient, but some prefer to adopt a half-reclining position on the couch, supporting themselves on the left forearm ; others manage best when standing by the couch with one foot raised to about the level of the seat of a chair.

I advise her to feel the pessary in position, following the rim with her finger as far as possible, and to note the loose rubber diaphragm, which may be wrinkled into folds ; some patients imagine that the pessary is much too large because of the looseness of the diaphragm, and need to be reassured on this point.

(*b*) I then ask her to remove the pessary herself by hooking her finger tip under the rim anteriorly or laterally, wherever she can reach best, and pulling on it.

I demonstrate, with a pessary in my hand, that the rim is easily compressed by pulling firmly on the rim and drawing the pessary through the small space between thumb and forefinger.

(*c*) When she has removed the pessary, I ask her to examine one in her hand; and I explain how the pessary fits inside the vagina, and point out the advantage of having the convex side uppermost, so that when the cap is invaginated by the protruding cervix the small gutter is formed round the rim.

Some authorities maintain that it is immaterial which side of the pessary is towards the cervix, but the patient herself readily appreciates the greater ease of removing the pessary when it is placed with the convex side towards the cervix.

(*d*) Now comes a most important part of the procedure—the exploration of the vaginal cavity and the identification of the cervix.

Patients with relatively short fingers may find some considerable difficulty in feeling the cervix; they can facilitate matters by bearing down to force the uterus downwards towards the examining finger. The patient should locate her cervix, so that she will know where to feel for it when the pessary is in position.

(*e*) The patient is next instructed in the actual procedure of inserting the pessary.

The pessary, suitably lubricated, as by being dipped into a solution of soapy water, should be held in the patient's right hand, with the rim compressed between thumb and fingers, and with the dome uppermost. (It is sometimes advisable, especially when there is a nervous spasm of the perivaginal muscles, to allow the patient to begin practising with a pessary of a smaller size than the size selected. The correct size can be substituted after she has succeeded in placing it correctly.) Then, in the squatting position and without reversing her hand, she should insert the rim through the introitus in a ***downward and backward direction***, following the lower curve of the posterior wall of the vagina.

The common error here is to push the pessary directly upwards, bringing it into contact with the projecting cervix. The rim may then slide over the cervix into the posterior fornix into its proper position; but more commonly it is directed forwards into the anterior fornix, when it presses the cervix towards the posterior wall, and leaves it uncovered and projecting between the posterior rim of the pessary and the vaginal wall (see Plate IV.).

I find it very helpful to emphasise the initial *downward* direction—" as if you are pushing it into the back passage "—explaining that this part of the rim will then slide upwards in a curved direction into its proper place, provided that it is kept in contact with the posterior vaginal wall.

If the patient makes this mistake of pushing the whole pessary into the anterior fornix, urge her to try to feel the uncovered cervix, and to feel that the cup of the pessary is empty. It is a good plan, especially where the cervix is low or unusually long, deliberately to put the pessary into the anterior fornix, so that the patient may feel the exposed cervix, and appreciate the discomfort of the projecting rim in front. She is then well warned against this error, which would render the pessary useless. It may be necessary to use a smaller size to demonstrate this error. Correctly fitted, the pessary is perfectly comfortable. Naturally, where a relatively small size is used there is sufficient extra room available for the cervix to be exposed posteriorly without any discomfort or projection of the rim anteriorly, and I regard this as one real and serious disadvantage of the smaller fitting. With the larger fitting, the discomfort and projection of the rim anteriorly make it obvious to the patient that the pessary is not properly adjusted.

I am emphasising this error because I believe it to be responsible for a number of the failures of the diaphragm pessary.

When the initial direction is correct the pessary will slide into the vagina, so that anteriorly the last portion of the rim to enter can be pushed up into the retro-pubic space, where it is supported by the pubic bone. The pessary then lies diagonally in the vagina and encloses the cervix.

(*f*) Confirming the correctness of the position of the pessary.

Finally I ask the patient to feel for the cervix through the thin rubber diaphragm, emphasising the importance of making sure that it is covered. This is often the only check possible to the patient, since she may be unable to reach the cervix if it has been pushed back into the posterior fornix, although it is in fact protruding into the vagina between the rim and the posterior vaginal wall, and is therefore not covered by the pessary.

The patient should then practise inserting and removing the pessary several times until she feels sufficiently confident. In most cases it is advisable that she should continue this practice at home, inserting the cap three or four times each day for a week; she should then return and insert the pessary for final inspection.

This may appear to be a cumbersome procedure, but it is my experience that it cannot be simplified without insecurity, except in exceptional cases.

Instructions for Fitting the Vault and Cervical Pessaries (Dumas, Prencap, Cercap, Racial, Unique, etc.).—The general procedure is the same as for the diaphragm pessary (see p. 78). *Again, I would urge the importance of teaching the patient to identify her cervix by digital exploration of her vagina, both before and after the pessary has been inserted.* She should check the proper adjustment of the pessary by making quite sure that the cervix is covered. In the case of pessaries with thin rubber domes (Racial and similar types, Prencaps and the small-fitting diaphragm pessaries), she will be able to feel the cervix through the thin rubber without dislodging the pessary; but with the Dumas and Unique pessaries, which have a relatively thicker dome, it will be necessary to tilt the pessary so that the finger can feel for the cervix within the pessary. When the cervix has been identified in this way, the pessary should be replaced by pushing it up to bring the rim again into contact with the vaginal vault or—in the case of cervical caps—with the base of the cervix. To insert these pessaries, they should be held in the same

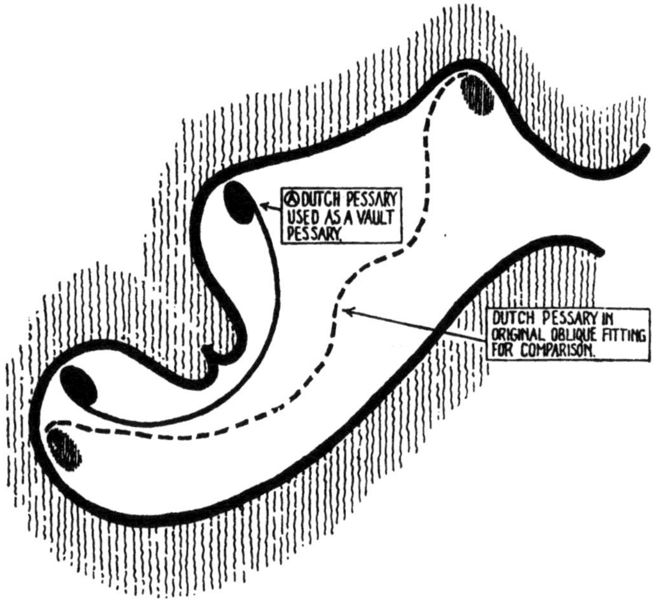

A. Alternative Method of Fitting a Diaphragm Pessary

The pessary is used as a vault pessary. A much smaller size is used than for the oblique fitting, as the anterior rim of the pessary rests in the anterior fornix instead of in the retro-pubic space, and the anterior vaginal wall is not covered by the rubber diaphragm.

In the illustration the pessary is placed with the concave side towards the cervix; in most cases the reverse position (convex side towards the cervix) is preferable.

way as the diaphragm pessary—the rim compressed between finger and thumb—but with the dome *downwards*, to bring the concave side of the pessary towards the cervix. The pessary must be pushed along the vagina and tilted over the cervix. The ease with which this is accomplished will, of course, depend upon the position and direction of the cervix. To remove the pessary the finger must be hooked over the rim at the front or side ; the pessary should then be tilted and drawn down and out of the vagina. Care should be taken to avoid dragging on the cervix and consequent strain on the uterine supports.

The Alternative Method of Fitting a Diaphragm (Dutch or Ramses) Pessary.—The diaphragm pessary can be used as a vault pessary, in which case much smaller sizes are fitted. For example, a patient who needs size 75 when the pessary is fitted in the original oblique position, so as to occlude the whole of the vaginal vault and also the anterior vaginal wall as far as the pubic bone, might need size 65 or 60 if the pessary is to be used as a vault pessary. In this latter position it is usually more satisfactory to fit the pessary concave side towards the cervix.

Comments on Choice of Size of Diaphragm Pessaries.—This difference in the two methods—oblique and vault—of fitting the Dutch or Ramses pessary almost certainly accounts for the difference in the sizes used by experienced gynæcologists. This discrepancy was revealed in discussions at the Seventh International Birth Control Conference, 1930.

Dr. Hannah Stone, of the New York Sanger Clinic, said :—

> " As to the size to be chosen, there seems to be a difference of opinion among clinicians in this respect. Some maintain that the pessary should fit circularly in the vagina, covering the cervix more like a cervical cap, and they select, accordingly, the smaller sizes, usually sizes 50 to 65. In my opinion, the diaphragm pessary is most satisfactory when it fits diagonally across the vagina, extending from the posterior fornix to the pubic bone in front. Hence, we generally choose the largest size which can comfortably be worn, the sizes usually ranging from 70 to 85 or even 90, varying with the depth of the vagina. Size 75 seems to be the most frequently prescribed."

Dr. Haire, referring to the original oblique fitting of the diaphragm pessary, remarked :—

> " . . . the hinder part of the pessary lies in the posterior fornix. The pessary lies almost longitudinally

in the vagina. In my opinion that pessary is too large as it lies there. I find with a great many women that if they cough or sneeze or make any other effort which increases their intra-abdominal pressure a force is produced which may dislodge one end of the pessary and make it lie absolutely longitudinally. I began by using the pessary in this way, and advocated it in my earlier writings, but since then I have come to use smaller pessaries."

On the same occasion Dr. J. H. Leunbach, Copenhagen, stated :—

" In the course of years I have arrived at the conclusion that large pessaries should be used—so large that they reach from the symphisis pubis up into the lacuna posterius vaginæ. And in far the greatest number of cases where I have seen a pessary fail, the pessary has been several numbers too small. For it has hitherto been the prevailing custom to use far too small sizes. It is still a ruling opinion that large pessaries should be avoided because they annoy. In my opinion this is wrong. The cases where the pessary annoys are more often those where it is too small and slips down in front."

Dr. Kaviöky (California) said :—

" Our . . . failures came mostly when we used smaller sizes and have diminished since we used large sizes . . ."

Dr. Antoinette Konikow, in " The Physician's Manual of Birth Control," p. 80, states :—

" In final position the front rim rests against the symphisis. The back part of the rim is behind and below the cervix in the posterior cul-de-sac and cannot be felt ; the cervix itself is usually felt far back, through the thin covering of the rubber. *The largest size which can be fitted comfortably should always be used.*"

Dr. Van de Velde (" Fertility and Sterility in Marriage," p. 330) also advises the large oblique fitting :—

" Of course, vital and motile sperms may quite possibly slip round the edge of the pessary, and enter the os. This was how the failures which have been observed in the use of the Mensinga, especially early in its history, when too little care was given to *exact fit*, and when only very small sizes were used. Since then we have learnt that the occlusive should be *as large as the vagina will permit. . . .*"

The results of a questionnaire to birth control clinics, quoted at the International Birth Control Conference, September, 1930, showed that at twenty-six American clinics (36,804 patients) the commonest sizes fitted were 70, 75 and 80. At sixteen British clinics (45,321 patients) the commonest sizes fitted were 70, 72½ and 75.

Of these forty-two clinics, the late Cromer Street Clinic in London (Dr. Norman Haire, Director), and the American Clinic at Reading, Pennsylvania, fit the smallest sizes, 10 mm. to 15 mm. smaller than the average for all.

I advise the original oblique fitting where possible, but in those cases where the retro-pubic space is absent the alternative vault fitting may be useful.

My further comments on fittings are :—

1. Where the small sizes are used, *i.e.*, as *vault pessaries*, there is more likelihood of the pessary's being wrongly placed—pushed into the anterior fornix, leaving the cervix exposed ; moreover, it is more easily dislodged during coitus. In addition, when the vagina is distended during coitus, there is less effective occlusion of the cervix and vault.

2. In the *oblique fitting* the size is determined by the size and length of the vagina and by the tone of the vaginal muscles.

There is no uniform relation between the size of the pessary and the age or number of children born. The average fittings are :—

Newly married	55 –70
Primipara	70 –75
Multipara	77½–82½

3. *The pessary is unsuitable or the size incorrect*, if :—

(*a*) The pessary slips out in front from under the pubic bone when the patient " bears down " ; or (*b*) Its presence in the vagina causes any pain or discomfort.

Although in nearly all cases I use the larger sizes in the oblique fitting, the patients almost without exception assure me, in reply to my routine question as to whether they can feel the pessary, that they " did not know it was there."

(*c*) There is any pain or discomfort to either partner during coitus; occasionally the husband is conscious of the rim.

(*d*) The pessary is found to be dislodged after coitus.

Contra-indications to the use of a diaphragm pessary include:—

1. *Cystocele and Rectocele.*—It may be possible to fit a diaphragm pessary which has some modification of the shape of the rim (as, for example, a Matrisalus), or to use the smaller vault fitting of the Dutch or Ramses pessary if there is sufficient support from the vaginal walls.

2. *Severe Chronic Constipation.*—The patient should be warned not to use the pessary when she finds, on vaginal examination, that the rectum is distended with fæces. The irregular bulging of the posterior vaginal wall, due to the distended rectum, will most probably prevent a satisfactory fit of the posterior part of the rim.

During occasional constipation, if coitus cannot be postponed, a sheath may be used as an alternative; or an additional protection in the form of jelly or suppository or tablet may be used.

3. *Laxity of the vaginal walls*, with insufficient tone to support the rim in the correct position.

4. *Prolapsus Uteri.*—The suitability or otherwise of a diaphragm pessary depends upon the degree of prolapse and the condition of the vaginal and perineal muscles. The pessary may act as a uterine support and thereby add to the comfort of the patient; or it may fail to retain its correct position within the vagina.

A ring pessary, worn to correct uterine prolapse, usually prevents a satisfactory fit of a diaphragm pessary. In some cases, however, the writer has found that a diaphragm pessary can be adjusted over the ring pessary, and the patient can be taught to remove the diaphragm without dislodging the ring. In other cases where this is not possible, the patient has been able to remove her ring pessary before inserting the diaphragm, and to replace the ring after removing the diaphragm.

5. *Absence of the retro-pubic* space from causes other than cystocele.

6. *Vaginal adhesions or tumours.*

7. *Inflammatory lesions with profuse muco-purulent discharge.*

8. *Intact Hymen.*—In cases where the hymen is poorly developed, however, and in cases where the patient has the hymen stretched or incised in preparation for the consummation of marriage, it is generally possible to fit a virgin with a diaphragm pessary on the eve of marriage. She should be warned that she will probably need a larger size in a month or two.

Spermicidal Lubricants Suitable for use with Occlusive Pessaries

Any contraceptive jelly or ointment, such as " G.P." ointment or Prentif jelly, may be used provided it does not contain a greasy base which is injurious to rubber (see p. 52). The consistency should be such that the lubricant adheres well to the rubber. " K.Y." jelly has excellent lubricating properties, but it is a very weak spermicide. It is preferable to combine good lubrication with effective spermicidal action. Patients vary in their individual reactions to the same preparation ; a jelly or ointment which proves satisfactory for one may be irritating for another.

When an occlusive pessary is used in combination with a contraceptive jelly or ointment, such as Mil-San jelly, the same jelly should be used as a lubricant for the rubber pessary.

CHAPTER V

METHODS OF CONTRACEPTION

TAMPONS AND SPONGES. THE DOUCHE

Tampons and Sponges.—Vaginal tampons of various materials were among the earliest known contraceptives. The oldest medical document, the Ebers papyrus, refers to the use of medicated grease or honey on lint.

Tampons and sponges act as vehicles for chemical spermicides, besides having mechanical action. Their main defect is that they are liable to be dislodged by the movements of the phallus and to leave the cervix exposed, unless they be so bulky as to be uncomfortable during coitus. Unless they are large enough to block the upper end of the vagina effectively, they may fail in their purpose.

Tampons of hydrophile cotton-wool, soaked in a spermicidal solution or smeared with jelly or ointment, appear to be acceptable and effective in certain cases. At the Zurich Conference, 1930, Dr. F. Mascaux said :—

> "After thirty years of contraceptive work in France and Belgium, I have reached the following conclusions : a simple wad of hydrophile cotton wool, soaked in vinegar or in lemon juice and applied to the cervix before coitus, is enough to prevent conception."

Sponges, usually combined with chemical contraceptives, have been widely used as mechanical contraceptives.

The spherical sponge, enclosed in a net with a string attachment to facilitate its removal, is usually too small and of the wrong shape. It is likely to be pushed into the posterior fornix during coitus, where it acts chiefly as a foreign body, but it may have some virtue on account of the spermicidal solution in which it has been soaked previously. As might have been expected from their size and shape, the small spherical sponges have not given good results.

Konikow, commenting on the inadequate protection afforded by the small " sanitary " sponges, remarks :—

> " . . . this method is entirely unsatisfactory. A large sponge which could not be displaced would interfere mechanically with intercourse."—(" Physician's Manual of Birth Control," by Antoinette F. Konikow, M.D., Ballière, Tindall & Cox, p. 71.)

The natural sea sponge is difficult to keep clean ; it will not stand repeated boiling. The fine grained rubber sponge is easier to clean and can be boiled.

The Racial Sponge is a large, flat fine-grained rubber sponge designed to cover the vaginal vault. It is made in two sizes, large and extra large, and is about ¾ inch thick. It is now being advised at the Mother's Clinic for Constructive Birth Control for those cases which are considered to be unsuitable for an occlusive pessary. Patients are instructed to soak the sponge in olive oil after first squeezing it in water, and then to press out the oil until the sponge is merely damp, when it is ready for insertion into the vagina. Patients are further instructed to wash out the sponge after use and then to boil it for two minutes in salt and water. It may be hung up to dry or stored in a covered jar of weak disinfectant. Its removal is advised in the morning or afternoon following coitus.

Stopes recommends the sponge as

> " the most suitable contraceptive for various types of cervical abnormality, either where the cervix is lacerated or proliferated, when the application of an occlusive cap is difficult or impossible. Also for cases where the cervix has been depressed or has been removed. If the uterus is not much prolapsed, the sponge is safe and satisfactory."—("Contraception," 3rd Edition, p. 163.)

When the patient can be fitted by a doctor and properly instructed, and provided that the vagina is suitable, I regard a diaphragm pessary as the method of choice in the pelvic conditions referred to by Dr. Stopes. The medicated sponge, as an alternative to the condom, may prove a useful contraceptive when the patient's pelvic condition negatives the use of any form of occlusive pessary or when she cannot obtain expert instruction and fitting, and when the condom is unacceptable. The sponge has the merit of simplicity and cheapness if it is used in conjunction with diluted vinegar, and of not requiring expert fitting and instruction in its use. At the same time, I think the best results would be obtained if the sponge were cut for each individual patient to fit the vaginal vault as neatly as possible. Some patients have found the Racial sponge unacceptable on account of its bulk; others complain that it tends to slip out of the vagina—a displacement most likely to occur in a multipara with stretched and weakened vaginal muscles and defective perineum.

"*Occlusator*" rubber sponges contain a central pocket for a chemical spermicide (suppository or tablet). These sponges in their present form are too small, and, like the natural "sanitary" sponges, are liable to be pushed up into the fornices, and to leave the cervix exposed during coitus.

Sponge used with Foam Powder.—Dr. De Vilbiss, Director of the Mothers' Health Clinics of Florida, has devised a method of using a rubber sponge as a reservoir for a contraceptive foam powder. The sponge, which measures $2 \times 2 \times \frac{3}{8}$ inches, is not intended necessarily to cover the cervical os or to remain *in situ*. The method is still in the experimental stage.

Cervical caps with sponge-covered domes are manufactured.

The Douche.—The douche, correctly administered, has primarily a mechanical action; its object is to distend the vagina sufficiently to open up the folds and furrows, and to flush out any semen which has not drained away, and any chemical residua (from suppositories, jellies or foaming tablets) and pent-up secretions.

It has, in addition, a definite spermicidal action. Clean tap water at body heat will immobilise sperms in ten seconds, so that a non-medicated water douche would appear to be as effective as most of the medicated douches in regard to spermicidal action. Nevertheless, it is customary to use medicated douches as part of a contraceptive method.

Post-coital douching alone is unreliable as a contraceptive measure, since those sperms which are deposited on the cervix may have reached the cervical canal before the solution enters the vagina, even though the douche be administered immediately after coitus. Moreover, the cervical mucus at the os, into which sperms may have been rubbed by the phallus during coitus, may be sufficiently tenacious to escape dislodgment during the irrigation of the vagina; and this mucus probably protects the spermatozoa from injury or destruction by the fluid.

For contraceptive purposes, douching may be advised in suitable cases :—

(*a*) *In Combination with other Methods.*—The douche, unless there are special reasons for advising otherwise, should be postponed until the following morning when coitus has taken place overnight.

With the commonly used combination of occlusive pessary, spermicidal lubricant and douche, the douche is delayed until the time for the removal of the pessary. The vagina should be irrigated with at least a pint of the fluid before the cervix is uncovered, and irrigated again after the removal of the pessary.

(*b*) *As an Emergency Measure.*—When a condom tears, or a pessary becomes dislodged during coitus, an immediate douche is advisable in the hope that, in this particular instance, the semen has not been ejaculated on to the cervix, so that all the spermatozoa are accessible to the action of the douche.

METHOD OF DOUCHING.—For contraceptive purposes the douche should be under pressure to distend the vagina sufficiently for the efficient irrigation of the whole of the vaginal cavity. The necessary pressure within the vagina may be obtained by regulating the outflow of fluid, and this can be done, irrespective of the woman's posture, by digital compression of the vulva around the bulb of the syringe, or by using the sliding shield supplied with the whirling spray type of syringe.

Distension of the vagina should be gradual, whether it is regulated by the pressure of the fluid in a douche-can or by the compression of the bulb of a syringe; and when sufficient pressure is reached the fluid should be released at the vulva.

To avoid excessive pressure, and with it the risk of forcing the fluid into the uterus and along the Fallopian tubes into the peritoneal cavity, the following precautions are advised by Dickinson and Bryant ("Control of Conception," p. 72):—

(*a*) The top of the fluid in the douche-can or -bag should not be more than 2 feet above the tip of the nozzle; or

(*b*) the bulb of the spray syringe should be compressed between thumb and finger only.

By this means they claim that the intra-vaginal pressure is kept within the safe limit of 60 to 80 mm. of mercury.

The experiments on animals of Carleton and Florey, and of Walton, suggest that there is probably no appreciable risk of harmful intra-vaginal pressure being attained, except in those cases where the cervix is so relaxed or damaged that the normal valve-like action of the internal os does not take place.

Position during Douching.—I disagree with the view that contraceptive douching can be effective only when the douche is administered with the woman in the recumbent position. Van de Velde ("Fertility and Sterility in Marriage," p. 353) states that:—

> "douching should take place *lying down*, *i.e.*, on a large bidet—the trunk should be supine, the legs parted, but not necessarily stretched."

The opposite view is expressed by Dickinson and Bryant ("Control of Conception," p. 72). They maintain that, with regulation of the outflow to secure adequate vaginal distension,

> "the douche can be used effectively to cleanse the cavity, with the woman seated. The reclining posture so often recommended for contraceptive douching is not needed, and, as a matter of fact, its field in local treat-

ment is the prolonged application of heat to inflamed, congested or sensitive areas."

SPERMICIDAL DOUCHES

Warm Water.—Plain water paralyses spermatozoa within a few seconds. It has the advantage of not introducing chemicals whose repeated use has yet to be proved harmless. Furthermore, there is the least likelihood of interference with the normal bacteriological vaginal flora.

Soapy Water.—For human sperms sodium oleate has a killing concentration of ½ per cent., which is equal to that of quinine and chinosol (Baker). An emulsion can be made quickly with soap flakes or powder; but patients should be warned not to use cheap brands of household soap on account of the irritating effects of the excess of alkali. A suitable solution may be prepared by adding to each quart of water about two-fifths of an ounce (roughly equivalent in volume to two of the ordinary large cubes of sugar) of a pure toilet soap, or two level tablespoonsful of Lux. This gives a solution of approximately 1 per cent. Hot water is necessary to make a satisfactory solution. After the use of a soapy douche, the syringe should be rinsed thoroughly with clear water to prevent the formation of a gelatinous deposit of soap within the syringe. Thousands of clinic patients are regularly using the soapy water douche in conjunction with an occlusive pessary, with no indication of irritation or other harmful effects.

Salt.—For the irrigation of the vagina, the concentration commonly used is one tablespoon of salt to the quart of warm water. Dickinson and Bryant point out that for rapid spermicidal effect, an 8 per cent. solution, that is, five tablespoons to the quart—is required.

Vinegar.—Two tablespoons to the quart of warm water gives an effective spermicidal concentration of acetic acid. Vinegar, which contains about 5 per cent. of acetic acid, is available in most households, and has the merit of cheapness; moreover, the solution is easily made.

Lemon Juice.—This is a convenient source of citric acid, and should be used at the same strength as the vinegar solution—two tablespoons to the quart.

Lactic Acid.—In a concentration of 1 drachm to the quart, this is useful in cases of leucorrhœa; but its spermicidal power is weak. A few patients find this strength irritating to the vaginal mucous membrane, and must use a weaker and therefore even less spermicidal solution.

Alum.—Half a drachm to the quart gives an astringent douche which is also an effective spermicide. I do not recommend it for regular use, except in cases where the vagina is unduly relaxed, or in cases of leucorrhœa with profuse secretion.

G.P.D. (douche).—This spermicidal solution contains ac. lactic, ac. citric and ol. pini pond. In the dilute form and in the presence of buffer proteins it has a *p*H value equivalent to that of the healthy vagina. It is especially indicated for post-coital douching in cases of leucorrhœa.

"Proseldis" Douching Pellets.—These contain zinc sulph., alum pot., ac. boric and chinosol.

GENERAL CONSIDERATIONS.—In combination with an occlusive rubber pessary, post-coital douching is the alternative to the use of a suppository, jelly or foam tablet, and is preferred by some patients for economic or hygienic reasons. When coitus takes place on retiring at the end of the day, douching should be postponed until the following morning, so as not to interfere with the post-coital sleep and rest. Only in exceptional cases, where the occlusive pessary should be removed within a short time after coitus, should the normal sequence of sexual intercourse be interrupted by the effort of douching overnight. I regard such interruption as so grave a drawback that I recommend some alternative method in such abnormal cases.

The douche has a further use as an emergency measure, immediately after coitus, when a defective condom has been used. It is also prescribed in conjunction with an occlusive pessary and chemical spermicide (suppository, tablet or jelly), when an additional safeguard is desirable.

CONTRA-INDICATIONS TO DOUCHING.—(*a*) *Absence of proper facilities*, due to overcrowding or travelling, lack of privacy and of the necessary materials and time for preparing and administering the douche.

(*b*) *Æsthetic Objections or Unpleasant Associated Symptoms.*—Douching causes some women to feel faint or exhausted, or to experience backache or pains in the limbs.

The argument that douching should be condemned on account of its interference with normal activity of the vaginal organisms does not apply in cases where chemical contraceptives are being regularly used. It is at least probable that a douche once or twice a week is beneficial in removing any chemical residue in these cases. The writer records a case of vaginitis, with profuse muco-purulent discharge, caused by accumulation within the vagina of the residue of cocoa-butter suppositories which had been used for several months. The patient was admitted to hospital, where the vaginal vault was found to be coated with a greasy deposit. There is ample clinical evidence that patients suffering from a mild leucorrhœa benefit from the contraceptive douche.

I am convinced of the contraceptive value of the post-coital douche used in conjunction with an occlusive pessary and spermicidal ointment or jelly. Clinic patients who have used this combined method successfully over periods long enough to establish its efficacy have become pregnant after omitting to douche.

Many patients prefer to douche for hygienic reasons. When there are objections to contraceptive douching, a chemical spermicide (jelly, suppository or tablet) may be substituted.

CHAPTER VI

METHODS OF CONTRACEPTION

THE CONDOM OR MALE SHEATH

THE condom is a thin sheath which is used during coitus to prevent contact between the seminal fluid and the vagina and cervix. It is unrolled over the erect penis before penetration, and, when properly used, the whole of the ejaculate is confined within the sheath and thus removed from the vagina when the phallus is withdrawn. It is, perhaps, the most widely used mechanical device; and, provided that it is properly tested before use, and is used with a chemical agent which acts both as a lubricant and a spermicide, it appears to be one of the most reliable contraceptives.

The condom has in the past been subjected to considerable disparagement in the literature on contraception. One of the main objections appears to be based on the assumption that the vagina absorbs certain substances from the seminal fluid, substances which have a beneficial effect on the woman's health. I have failed to discover any scientific evidence that this is so; but, even should this prove to be the case, it may still be that the advantages of the sheath outweigh its disadvantages, and that it compares very favourably with other methods of contraception. I am of the opinion that many of the objections to the sheath are due to its improper use—sensation impaired by unnecessarily thick rubber or by a bad fit (too loose or too tight), failures due to the use of defective sheaths or to delay in adjusting the sheath, etc. Where the sheath is properly used and proves acceptable to both partners, the sex life appears to be perfectly satisfactory. It is a significant fact that the sheath remains the method of choice of a large proportion of married people.

Condoms are made from rubber (cut-sheet rubber, rubber solution and latex) and from animal membrane—so-called "skin" sheaths. *Skin condoms* have the advantage of extreme thinness, so that in use they are practically imperceptible; but they are more liable to perforations than are rubber condoms, and they need extreme care in handling, and have to be damped before or after adjusting. Moreover, on a commercial scale they cannot be tested satisfactorily by inflation. *Rubber condoms* are of varying thicknesses. A very thin rubber condom is not necessarily less strong than a thicker one, and has the great advantage that it interferes less with sensation. The washable thick rubber sheaths can be used several times, provided that due care is exercised. Patients are sometimes advised that such sheaths can be used half a dozen times, but in fact they are generally used more than this. In one case on record the same washable sheath was used regularly for a period of eighteen months. Rubber sheaths are elastic, and can be tested for reliability on a commercial scale by inflation. The elasticity is an advantage in securing a satisfactory fit within limits, but a sheath which is too small and is therefore unduly stretched causes discomfort and may constrict the urethra painfully. Sheaths are usually made in three sizes—small, medium and large. Unlike the skin sheaths, the rubber sheaths can be rolled, and are therefore easier to adjust.

Rubber Condoms and Washable Sheaths

As rubber may deteriorate somewhat rapidly, *sheaths should bear the date of manufacture* with a warning against their use after a specified period from that date, *or the date after which they should not be used.* Users should also be warned not to lubricate washable sheaths with vaseline or with greasy ointments or creams, or to use them repeatedly in conjunction with cocoa-butter or cocola suppositories, since grease in any form is harmful to rubber.

The sheath should be used in conjunction with a spermicidal lubricant, which should be made up in a non-fatty base such as glycerite of starch or tragacanth. G.P. jelly

(Gilmont Products) and Prentif lubricating jelly are suitable lubricants. About half a teaspoonful of the lubricant should be placed inside the tip of the sheath before it is unrolled over the phallus ; and the outside of the sheath should be lubricated with the minimum amount necessary to prevent soreness of the vagina. An alternative procedure is to exclude air from the free space (the teat end or about ½ inch at the end of the plain end) by squeezing, before unrolling the sheath over the phallus, and to lubricate the outside of the sheath only. This is preferable if there is any tendency for the sheath to slip off during coitus. Free lubrication will facilitate the consummation of marriage ; afterwards, if the vaginal secretions are normal, it may prove a disadvantage, as excessive lubrication may seriously diminish sexual sensation during coitus. A small space, from which most of the air is excluded, should be left at the end of the sheath to make room for the ejaculate, and for the greater comfort of the wearer. This space is provided in the teat-ended type of sheath.

If the sheath is found after use to be perfect, and if the directions given on p. 103 are followed, complete security is assured by these means. If the sheath breaks, or if there is a flaw in the rubber which permits the escape of sperms, the use of the spermidical lubricant lessens somewhat the risk of conception ; but additional safety can be secured by the insertion into the vagina shortly before coitus of a chemical spermicide (suppository, tablet or jelly).

If a defect in the sheath is detected after coitus immediate measures should be taken by the use of a douche, or of a spermicidal jelly which acts immediately, to immobilise and destroy any sperms which are within the vagina.

In spite of all precautions, there is always a possible risk of conception when a sheath is defective, since sperms may be ejaculated directly into the cervical canal, and out of reach of spermicides or douches. IT IS THEREFORE OF FIRST IMPORTANCE TO USE DATED SHEATHS OF RECENT MANUFACTURE AND GOOD QUALITY AND TO EXAMINE THEM CAREFULLY IMMEDIATELY BEFORE AND AFTER USE.

Inflation is the best test of the strength of the material ;

and a rubber condom of good quality should also stretch lengthways about a yard without tearing. It should always be carefully examined before use, and its adequacy should be tested again immediately after use by half filling it with water or by inflating it with air, and then pressing it firmly from the top to detect any leakage.

Directions for the use of the Rubber Sheath

1. *The sheath should be tested for defects* immediately before use. The presence of a flaw or tear in the rubber can be determined by distending the sheath with air (blowing into it) or with water (filling it three parts full and compressing from the top). The outside of the sheath should be quite dry before the water test.

2. *The sheath should be rolled before use and adjusted by unrolling it over the erect penis.* An attempt to draw on an unrolled sheath may tear the rubber.

3. *Spermicidal jelly* (about half a teaspoonful) should be placed inside the tip of the sheath immediately before it is unrolled over the phallus. The outside of the sheath may then be lubricated with the jelly.

Alternatively, air should be excluded from the teat end of the sheath by squeezing, or a space of about ½ inch from which the air has been excluded should be left at the tip of the plain end sheath ; and the outside of the sheath only should be lubricated (see list of suitable lubricants, p. 104).

4. *The sheath should be adjusted before any penetration takes place,* even though ejaculation is not intended in the preliminary coitus. Conception may occur through fertilisation by one of the sperms which may be present in the pre-ejaculatory secretion.

5. *Withdrawal should take place before full detumescence* to avoid exudation of seminal fluid at the base of the sheath. Sperms deposited at the vulva may succeed in finding their way into the womb, and there are records of pregnancy resulting in this manner.

6. *A new sheath should be used for a subsequent coitus,* even though a second ejaculation is not intended. If a washable sheath is in use, it should be removed, thoroughly washed

and readjusted before commencing the subsequent coitus. A preliminary cleansing of the penis may fail to remove or kill all the spermatozoa which are present, and the mucus which continues to ooze from the urethra may contain active spermatozoa.

7. *The sheath should be examined for defects immediately after use* to avoid delay in taking the secondary measures for the prevention of conception if these are indicated.

8. *Facilities for douching or inserting a spermicide* after the removal of the sheath should be available for use in case the sheath tears during use. Even when a spermicide has already been used in addition to the sheath as a second line of defence, the use of a further supply of spermicide immediately after coitus will lessen still more the risk of failure. PermFoam or Mil-San jellies, which act immediately and independently of vaginal moisture, are effective spermicides for this purpose.

9. Drying and powdering is the most satisfactory method of preserving washable sheaths. *When not in use, washable sheaths should be kept unrolled, thoroughly dry and powdered inside and outside with French chalk, in a cool, dry atmosphere not exposed to light.* They should not be carried for any length of time in pockets, exposed to the warmth of the body ; and they should not be placed unwrapped in pyjama pockets in contact with soiled handkerchiefs.

> *Note.*—To reduce to a minimum the risk of failure, I advise the routine use of a chemical spermicide (jelly, tablet or suppository) to be inserted into the vagina before coitus, in addition to the use of the sheath by the husband.

SPERMICIDAL LUBRICANTS suitable for use with rubber sheaths :—

Contraceptaline.
Durol.
" G.P." Jelly.
Prentif Jelly.
Prentif Spermicidal Compound.
Mil-San Jelly.

Note.—" K.Y." jelly has an excellent consistency as a lubricant, but its spermicidal power is probably negligible.

Skin Condoms

Skin Condoms are made from the peritoneal coverings of the bowels of animals (sheep, calf, goat). Skin condoms are not elastic and cannot be rolled. In use, they need to be secured at the base with tape or rubber band. The slight stiffness of texture can be removed by the application of a contraceptive jelly lubricant. Moistening a skin condom with a damp sponge will soften it, and this measure is sometimes adopted in order to secure a comfortable fit. Unlike rubber, this membrane is not damaged by vaseline or by greasy creams.

A skin condom should be tested before use by distension with air or water, as in the case of the rubber condom. If the skin condom fits closely, it is best to leave a small space at the tip to receive the ejaculate ; usually, however, the looseness of the fit renders this unnecessary. The usual lubrication with a spermicidal jelly is recommended.

After use the condom should be cleaned at once with soap and water if it is to be reserved for future use.

It may be preserved in water or alcohol, or coated with liquid vaseline ready for use.

The Acorn Condom (or American tip) is a short sheath made to fit over the glans penis alone. There is little demand for this type ; it has no advantage over the normal type and is less reliable.

The Feminine Sheath, or " Capote Anglaise," is a large rubber or " skin " sheath with an inflated rim, which is worn as a lining to the vagina. When in use it resembles the condom in preventing direct contact between the phallus and the vagina, and in forming an effective barrier between the spermatozoa and the cervical os. It is rarely used.

Advantages of the Condom.—1. Simplicity of technique.

2. It can be used for the consummation of marriage, where the bride is a virgin, and during the first month of

marriage, when the vagina and introitus are insufficiently stretched to allow the painless adjustment of an occlusive pessary.

3. Where there is a tendency to premature ejaculation, the slight diminution of sensation which results from wearing a sheath may be an advantage.

4. Its efficacy can be tested immediately after use. The anxiety due to lack of absolute confidence in other methods of contraception must persist until the time of the next menstrual period.

5. For the many women with sexual inhibitions which result in acute distaste for the manipulations involved in using an occlusive pessary, or in douching, the sheath may prove the only acceptable contraceptive method.

6. The sheath is particularly useful when the wife is unable to consult a doctor personally to be fitted with an occlusive pessary and instructed in its use.

7. It can be advised for those cases in which local pelvic conditions preclude the use of an occlusive pessary.

8. The efficacy of the sheath is not affected by constipation nor by variations in the vaginal secretions.

9. The sheath is a protection against venereal disease contagion during sexual intercourse.

Disadvantages of the Condom.—1. Impairment of sensation. The sensitive nerve endings around the corona of the glans are cut off from the normal contact with the vagina. Gasoline rubber, of which material some sheaths are made, is a poor conductor of heat, and this defect causes further impairment of sensation, and, to some people, definite discomfort. The latex sheath, which is extremely thin and a good conductor of heat, causes the minimum interference with sensation.

2. Delay and interference with the normal sequence of coitus at a stage when this is least tolerable.

3. The adjustment of the sheath causes erection to subside in some cases.

4. Increased friction, due to lack of the male pre-ejaculatory secretions, may cause soreness of an abnormally dry vagina. This can be remedied by proper lubrication.

5. If in normal coitus the woman benefits from the absorption of elements of the male semen by the vaginal mucous membrane, then by depriving her of this contact the sheath is physiologically imperfect.

POSSIBLE CAUSES OF FAILURE.—1. *A defective sheath.* —The rubber of sheaths which have been stored for some months may have perished. As previously stated, only *dated* and tested sheaths of good quality should be used, and the sheaths should be tested immediately before and after use.

2. *Delay in the adjustment of the condom until just before ejaculation,* so that the pre-ejaculatory mucus, which may contain active sperms, reaches the vagina. Living sperms have been found in the secretion which appears at the urethral orifice of the erect penis before ejaculation occurs.

3. *A second intromission after the removal of the sheath* without the protection of a new sheath or the same sheath properly cleansed, although a second ejaculation does not occur. Spermatozoa in the pre-ejaculatory secretion may effect conception.

4. *Neglect to withdraw the penis until after the erection has partially or completely subsided.* The consequent looseness of the fit may enable the semen to ooze out from the base of the sheath into the vagina or upon the vulva. In extreme cases the whole condom itself may be left within the vagina.

RELIABILITY.—Clinic records of the methods tried before visiting the clinic show a fairly high percentage of failures, but it must be remembered that these cases represent a selected class, and in most cases there is evidence that proper care has not been taken. Where the sheath is being used successfully and is giving satisfaction, the woman would not apply to the clinic.

Under the auspices of the Birth Control Investigation Committee, an analysis has been made of three sets of data, covering nearly 1,000 cases and derived from :—

1. Replies (432) to a questionnaire sent out by the B.C.I.C. to women who applied for it.

2. Replies collected by a private clinic.

3. A series of visitors' reports on patients of a clinic.

In the analysis, a method which has been used continuously for at least a year without an unwanted pregnancy is regarded as successful.

The sheath, with one or more adjuncts, was successful in 98 per cent. of cases, the sheath alone in 82 per cent. of cases.

CHAPTER VII

METHODS OF CONTRACEPTION

INTRA-UTERINE CONTRACEPTIVES

1. Those which have a part of the device within the cervical canal and projecting into the vagina.
   Vagino-uterine stem pessaries.
2. Those which are entirely within the uterine cavity.
   Uterine stars and rings.

1. **Vagino-uterine Stem Pessaries.**—For over fifty years various forms of intra-uterine stems have been in use. They all suffer from the grave disadvantage of keeping open a channel of infection from vagina to uterus. They are also liable to cause injury by mechanical pressure or by irritation.

Walton[1] and Carleton and Florey[2] have shown that the external os in rabbits and dogs appears to act as an efficient valve, allowing free drainage from the uterus into the vagina, but preventing the ingress, even during coitus, of substances from the vagina.

Drawbacks and Dangers.—Clinical results appear to justify the misgivings of those who foretold dangers and disadvantages from the use of such vagino-uterine appliances. There is considerable variation in the shape and size of the cervical canal and uterine cavity, both in primiparæ and in multiparæ, and mechanical injuries inflicted by the insertion of an appliance which is not well adapted to the size and shape of the uterine canal of the individual patient have not infrequently occurred. In addition, trauma has resulted from the pressure or the irritation of ill-fitting appliances and from the breaking of an appliance *in situ.*

[1] A Walton, "On the Function of the Rabbit Cervix during Coitus," *Brit. Journ. of Obstet. & Gynæcol.*, 1931, XXVII.
[2] H. M. Carleton and Howard Florey, "Birth Control Studies," *Brit. Journ. of Obstet. & Gynæcol.*, 1931, XXXVIII.

Acute inflammation of the uterus and adnexa has frequently arisen, owing to direct infection from vaginal organisms, and several deaths are recorded.

The following is a list of records of 381 deaths and disorders due to the use of stem pessaries, collected by Reist and quoted by Dickinson and Bryant (" Control of Conception," p. 112) :—

Deaths from general peritonitis or sepsis		17
(Includes 8 in which stems were deliberately introduced to produce abortion.)		
Endometritis with fever		75
Purulent inflammations of adnexa or parametritis		70
Septic abortions from presence of stems		62
Irregular bleedings		60
Peritonitis : general 38, pelvic 6		44
Uterine colic		28
Abscess in cervix or corpus		12
Perforations		9
Into uterine wall	5	
Into anterior vaginal wall	1	
Into bladder	1	
Into rectum	1	
Into cul-de-sac of Douglas	1	

Nordmeyer (*Dtsch. med. Wschr.*, November 27th, 1936) reports various pathological effects, mostly requiring extensive operative treatment, which resulted from the use of intra-uterine pessaries.

Contraceptive Evaluation of Stem Pessaries.—Of over 100 failures recorded, the large majority ended in abortion, mostly with septic complications. There is evidence of possible injury to the developing embryo.

2. **The Intra-uterine (Gräfenberg) Ring.**—This appliance differs in an important respect from the stem pessaries, since it is placed ***entirely within the uterus***, so that no part projects beyond the inner os if the ring is of correct size. In this way the danger of ascending infection from the vagina is avoided.

The object of the method is to produce a *revocable* sterility, but a sterility extending over long periods of several months or years.

Over ten years ago, Dr. Ernst Gräfenberg, of Berlin, began inserting into the uterus a silkworm-gut star, with one of the silk ends projecting through the cervical canal to facilitate removal. There was the usual drawback of cervico-uterine methods (bacterial invasion of the uterus), and the projecting end was uncomfortable for the husband. He therefore abandoned this method in favour of the purely intra-uterine form, using first the silkworm-gut star, then the ring of silkworm-gut covered with fine silver wire, and finally rings of gold or silver wire twisted spirally. He uses five sizes varying from 1·5 cm. to 3 cm. in diameter (1·75 cm. for average-sized uterus).

Gräfenberg, at the Zurich Conference, 1930, described fully his intra-uterine method.

Selection of Size of Ring and Preparation of uterus.—He ascertains the position and size of the uterus and the width and elasticity of the cervical canal by passing a uterine sound, taking the usual aseptic precautions. It is often necessary to dilate the cervix with Hegar dilators, Nos. 5 and 6. A cervix which admits Hegar No. 6 is sufficiently dilated to admit the ring and introducer.

Introduction of the Ring.—A selection of different sized rings, sterilised by boiling, is kept in readiness. The pliable silver ring, of such a size as entirely to fill the uterine cavity without protruding into the cervical canal, is then introduced into the uterine cavity. The special introducer resembles a uterine sound with a notched extremity. The pliable ring is compressed as it enters the cervix, but returns to its original circular form in the uterine cavity. Gräfenberg observes that it is most important that the introducer be pushed upwards until it reaches the dome of the uterus, after which the introducer is withdrawn, and the ring remains in position, being "pulled off the fork by contact with the walls of the uterus."

According to Gräfenberg, an anæsthetic is rarely necessary, as the operation is practically painless.

Removal of the Ring.—To remove the ring, the uterine

sound is inserted, again with the usual aseptic precautions, and the ring located. It is then pulled through the cervix with long polypus forceps or with a specially designed hooked instrument.

Formerly Gräfenberg removed and replaced the ring once a year. Now he leaves the ring *in situ* indefinitely, provided that the generative organs remain healthy and the ring in good position. The position of the ring can be verified by the use of the sound or by X-ray examination.

To quote from his own paper :—

> [1] " The insertion of the ring is followed by slight bleeding for the first few days. It is easily understood that superficial lesions of the mucous membrane may occur during the introduction of the ring. These lesions ooze blood and mucus until the epithelial layer has grown again. Frequently, uterine contractions also occur, giving rise to discomfort similar to menstrual pains. The dilatation itself causes some pain, which can last for several hours, but the contractions soon cease, and there is no further sensitiveness after one or two days.
>
> " It is most important to watch the patient's temperature, because bacteria may penetrate through the lesions in the uterine mucosa. The patient's temperature should therefore be taken regularly for the first three days. I examine my patients at the end of the first week, and after the first menstruation. The first examination is important so that the presence of any inflammation may be determined in time, and the second because the first menstruation following the insertion is often accompanied by very heavy bleeding and the ring might be expelled at the time. The presence of the ring may, therefore, be verified at this examination. Later, the risk of losing it is less, and the patient then waits a year before returning for a re-examination.
>
> " These symptoms occur only during the first weeks ; later, the patient has no further trouble. Only if these symptoms persist should the ring be removed, and then re-inserted after a certain length of time."

To avoid the risk of inserting a ring into a pregnant uterus, Gräfenberg advises that it should be inserted only immediately after a menstrual period, and it should not be inserted within six weeks after a confinement.

[1] " An Intra-uterine Contraceptive Method," by Dr. Ernst Gräfenberg. *Proceedings of Seventh International Birth Control Conference*, September, 1930. " Practice of Contraception," p. 33.

CONTRA-INDICATIONS TO THE USE OF THE INTRA-UTERINE RING.—1. *Any acute or chronic inflammation or infection of the pelvic organs.*

A history of former pelvic inflammation is an indication for special care, because of the danger that the intra-uterine manipulation may cause an old infection to light up. Gräfenberg emphasises the need for the thorough preliminary gynæcological examination by an experienced gynæcologist, the examination to include a bacteriological test of the genital secretions, and, if necessary, a blood-fixation test for gonorrhœa in doubtful cases.

Subsequent infections, or the lighting up of an old infection, necessitate the immediate removal of the ring.

2. *Menorrhagia.*

3. *Sub-mucous fibroids of fundus or cervix.*

Gräfenberg does not regard as contra-indications :—

1. Tumours (excluding sub-mucous fibroids of fundus or cervix).
2. Infantile uterus.
3. Simple cervical catarrh without hyperæmia.

Extract from letter from Gräfenberg, dated October 14th, 1932

" I have only slightly altered my method since Zurich.

" As the simple silver rings are sometimes difficult to extract and lose their shape, I usually only use those with a silk ring within the spiral.

" With women inclined to hæmorrhage I prefer a ring made out of gold wire rather than silver. These rings I also allow to remain still longer. I convince myself, after one year, that all is in order, and then leave them two to three years in the womb."

Physiological and Pathological Action of the Ring.—Gräfenberg has no record of the development of uterine cancer in his ten years' experience of this method, although many of his patients have reached the cancer age. He has ample evidence that the ring does not cause permanent sterility; in fact, he has had numerous cases of pregnancy occurring immediately after removal of the ring. He claims that the hypoplastic, infantile uterus is stimulated by the ring to develop normally, and that the presence of the ring in such a case acts as a cure for scanty and irregular menstruation and for dysmenorrhœa. He has never seen any cases of permanent damage to the uterine mucosa or to the uterine muscles.

Microscopic examination by Gräfenberg and Professor Robert Mayer, of Berlin, of curettings from uteri which had contained the ring for one or more years showed no inflammatory changes, but a hyper-decidual condition of the mucosa was always observed. Gräfenberg believes that this condition of the endometrium causes sterility by preventing the embedding of a fertilised ovum. He regards the possibility of malignant growth arising as a result of the irritation of the foreign body in the uterus as remote because " the mucous membrane in which a growth might be liable to appear is thrown off every month and replaced by a new one."

On the other hand, Stefko and Lourie, who have described a similar condition of the endometrium, regard the condition as pathological. They found a constant marked decrease of the *p*H of the uterine secretions, and suggest that the spermicidal power of these acid secretions accounts for the contraceptive action of the ring. It is a clinical fact, however, that both fertilisation and embedding of the ovum can occur, and Gräfenberg himself says that the ring does not prevent tubal pregnancy.

Evidence is steadily accumulating of the danger of this intra-uterine method of contraception, and even in the hands of gynæcological specialists, who are aware of the contra-indications to its use, acute pelvic conditions have resulted.

In one case a ring which had been in the uterus twelve months was found to be embedded in the uterine wall; and when gouged out with a curette, was found to have pieces of uterine muscle adherent to it.—(Dr. Trevor B. Davies, letter to *Brit. Med. Journ.*, January 4th, 1932.)

In Germany, according to W. Kolde (*Zentralbl. f. Gynäk.*, April 23rd, 1932) gynæcologists have expressed a general condemnation of the insertion into the uterus of a silk or silver ring for purposes of birth control.

Carleton publishes the results of experiments on rabbits

and monkeys (chapter on the Pathology of Contraception in "The Chemical Control of Conception," Chapman and Hall, 1935). In the breeding experiments, he found that rings and spirals of silver, gold or nickel, rubber-covered rings and many other foreign bodies were effective contraceptives "provided that they occupied the greater length of the uterine cavity." Histological observations of the uterine mucosa, made from four months onwards after insertion of a *silver* uterine ring, showed the following pathological changes: "(1) flattening of the uterine mucosa and obliteration of the glands due to pressure of the ring against the endometrium; (2) a variable degree of endometritis; (3) the presence of innumerable small, dark brown granules—mostly extra-cellular—in the corium." The granules were found to be silver sulphide, and the ring itself in such cases is black and brittle, owing to the formation of silver sulphide. Blackened and sulphided rings have been removed from human uteri, and the presumption is that a condition of localised argyria existed in these human uteri. Dr. Carleton emphasises the possible carcinogenic effect of a silver ring in the fundus uteri. He concludes: "All the evidence to hand points to the method as one to be condemned."

Effect of the Intra-uterine Ring in situ *during Pregnancy.*—Gräfenberg recommends the removal of the ring, followed by curettage of the uterus, in cases of pregnancy. It would appear from the records of failures with the Gräfenberg ring that the uterus is remarkably tolerant of the presence of this foreign body; spontaneous abortion does not occur in all cases, and a pregnancy is not always terminated by the manipulation involved in removal of the ring.

Norman Haire reports a case of a pregnancy which continued to term in the presence of the intra-uterine ring. This patient desired the child, and refused to have the ring removed. He says:—

> "I kept the woman under regular and frequent observation during the whole of the pregnancy, and had her X-rayed four times. . . . The patient had an uneventful and normal pregnancy, and I confined her

> myself with Somnifaine anæsthesia on February 8th, 1931. She was a primipara, aged 25. Labour began at 2.30 a.m. At 8.25 a.m. the ring came out of the vagina during a pain. On examination, I found the os fully dilated and the membranes unruptured. These were ruptured by hand at 8.40 a.m. and the child was born at 9.10 a.m. It cried immediately, and on examination was found to be quite normal. The placenta was born ten minutes later. The puerperium was uneventful. Mother and child are quite well."—(" International Medical Group for the Investigation of Contraception," 4th Issue, p. 6.)

Sjövall (*Zentralbl. f. Gynäk.*, November 4th, 1933) reports the spontaneous delivery at term of a normal child, which was closely preceded by expression of a silver intra-uterine pessary which the patient herself had introduced two years previously with the aid of an illuminated speculum and removed during the menses. He states that if pregnancy should follow the insertion of an intra-uterine pessary, abortion during the early months usually occurs, but that not a few cases have been reported in which both the contraceptive pessary and the fœtus have been delivered at or near term, the latter sometimes showing marks of injury by the former.

Van de Velde does not take an optimistic view of pregnancy with the ring in the uterus. He states :—

> " If an abortion occurs, as is generally the case, the resultant complications are even more serious than usual ; and, if pregnancy goes to term, the ring must have injurious effects on the child."—(" Fertility and Sterility in Marriage," 1931, p. 358.)

I have been unable to discover any record of association of the ring with abnormal development of the fœtus, although a case is reported of a nine to ten weeks' pregnancy where the ring was found to be " embedded in the corion, and was presumably responsible for the pain, discharge and fever. The fœtus appeared normal. . . ."—(Colonel Green Armytage, letter to *Brit. Med. Journ.*, Jan. 2nd, 1932.)

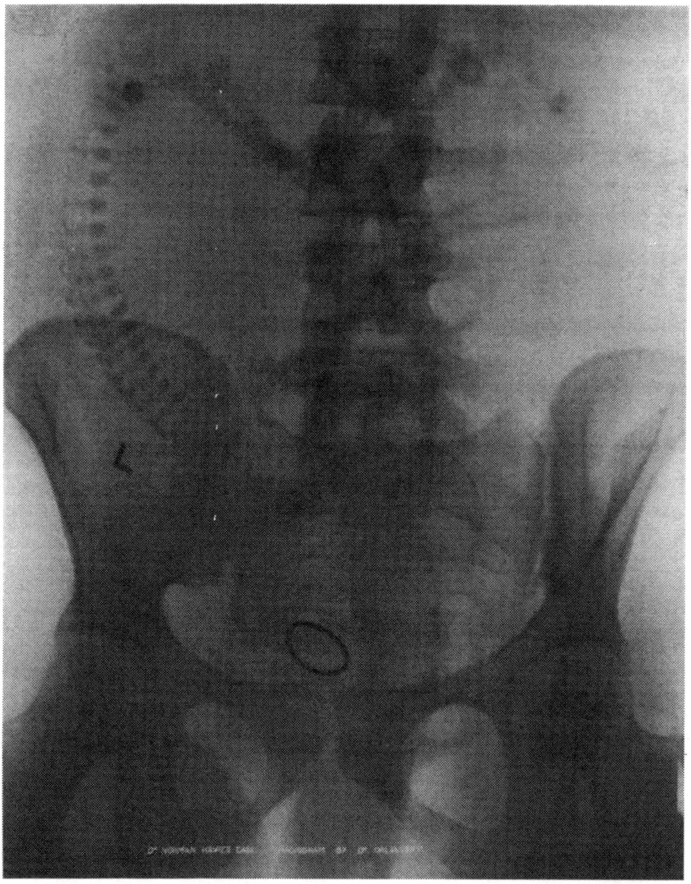

PREGNANCY WITH RING *IN SITU*

(*Reproduced by courtesy of Dr. Norman Haire.*)

[*To face p.* 116.

Clinical Results

Gräfenberg reported (Zurich, 1930) that he had fitted the following intra-uterine devices :—

400 silkworm-gut stars . . } 1,100 silkworm-gut rings . }	3·1 per cent. failures.
600 silver rings . . .	1·6 per cent. failures.

He has never claimed that the method is 100 per cent. successful.

Dr. J. H. Leunbach, of Copenhagen, inserted rings into 175 patients during a period of nine months ending May, 1930, with nine failures (more than 5 per cent. of failures in less than a year). He concludes that the method is neither sufficiently reliable nor sufficiently harmless to justify further experiment, and has therefore abandoned it.

His results are summarised below :—

175 *Women fitted*—
- 71 *satisfactory* cases—ring in place, 69,
  ring removed because pregnancy desired, 2.
- 95 *unsatisfactory* cases—
  - 35 (20 per cent.) spontaneously expelled (5 pregnant).
  - 4 pregnancies with ring *in situ*.
  - 49 rings removed on account of bleeding, discharge or pain.
  - 7 rings to be removed for same reason.
  - 3 rings removed because of gonorrhœa.
  - 1 ring inserted by mistake during pregnancy.
  - 6 patients lost touch with.

Dr. Helena Wright had, since July, 1930, inserted rings in 38 patients during a period of seventeen months. Her results are summarised below :—

38 *Women fitted* (46 rings inserted)—
- 36 for contraception,
- 2 for sterility.

10 *satisfactory fittings*—including three re-insertions after spontaneous expulsions.
36 *unsatisfactory* fittings—
33 spontaneous expulsions (approx. 70 per cent.).
1 removal, on account of hæmorrhage.
1 removal, followed by hysterectomy on account of severe sepsis.
1 removal for prophylactic reasons.

In May, 1932, only 8 of her 39 patients still had the rings.—(" Medical Problems of Contraception," *Brit. Med. Journ.*, June 4th, 1932.)

However, her conclusions differ from those of Leunbach. She states :—

> " The results in the 9 cases where rings have been retained are so good, and the patients so intensely appreciative, that I am encouraged to persevere."—(" International Medical Group for the Investigation of Contraception," 4th Issue, p. 65.)

She proposes to insert rings in suitable cases provided that the patient will practise continuously some other contraceptive method during the first trial year.[1]

Dr. Norman Haire, in a period of two years, has fitted over 400 intra-uterine rings, of which number just over half were for clinic patients. He inserts a ring during menstruation, and replaces it once a year, using nitrous oxide anæsthesia for nervous patients.

He now advises the additional use of a contraceptive tablet or suppository. For menorrhagia following the insertion of the ring, he prescribes cotarnine tablets. He claims that in the majority of cases the ring does not exert any noticeable effect on menstruation. He emphasises that the ring should only be inserted by a skilled gynæcologist.

[1] In a personal communication (November, 1936), Dr. Wright states that subsequent clinical results have not been encouraging, and that she now discourages patients from trying the intra-uterine ring. She inserts the ring " only if the patient insists in spite of knowing the disadvantages of the method."

He gives me the following analysis, prepared in 1931, of the results of his first 400 cases :—

In 20 per cent. the ring came out.

In $3\frac{1}{2}$ per cent. pregnancy followed as a result of the ring coming out.

In 6 per cent. one had to come to the conclusion that the woman could not keep the ring in. He writes : " I now find that I can get any woman to retain a ring if I choose a suitable size and consistency."

In 5 per cent. of cases pregnancy took place in spite of the ring being in position.

He states :—

" Of the catastrophic complications which are supposed by many critics to be an inevitable consequence of the use of this method, I have had no experience. . . . Many of my patients have been wearing the ring for over two years, and the greater my experience with the method the more I am convinced of its value in suitable cases."—(" International Medical Group for the Investigation of Contraception," 4th Issue, p. 69.)

Conclusions.—The following points indicate the limitations and dangers of the intra-uterine ring method :—

1. The selection of suitable cases involves the skill and experience of a gynæcological specialist.
2. Acute and dangerous complications are probable if :—
   (*a*) The ring is inserted in a patient whose vagina, uterus and tubes are not perfectly healthy.
   (*b*) A subsequent infection or inflammatory condition develops. Hence the patient must be under constant supervision by the gynæcologist so that the ring may be removed immediately if trouble develops.
   (*c*) The patient has a past history of pelvic sepsis. And old latent infection may light up.
3. The method is not 100 per cent. successful : pregnancy may occur in spite of the presence of the ring in the uterus.

4. In a large number of cases, the ring is ejected by the uterus, often without the knowledge of the patient.

A guarantee of its presence in the uterus at any particular moment involves either identification by insertion of a uterine sound, or a radiographic examination of the pelvis.

5. The ring may have to be removed on account of pain or irregular and profuse hæmorrhage.

6. There is now experimental evidence in support of the possibility of a carcinogenic effect of a *silver* ring on the uterus.

CHAPTER VIII

OTHER METHODS OF CONTRACEPTION

Coitus Interruptus

COITUS interruptus, or withdrawal of the penis from the vagina immediately before the male orgasm, in order that ejaculation may take place outside the vagina, is a primitive and still widespread method of contraception. From records at the Walworth Clinic of methods previously tried, it would appear to be by far the commonest, and at the same time the most unreliable method in use by the clinic type of patient; and the patient's faith in the efficacy of the method is gradually shattered by a steady increase in the size of her family.

CAUSES OF FAILURES.—1. Premature emission.

2. Presence of normal spermatozoa in the pre-ejaculatory secretion. In 24 specimens examined by Dr. Abraham Stone, sperms were found in 5:

3. Second coitus without effective cleansing of the penis (re-entry after ejaculation).

4. Motile sperms, from semen deposited on the vulva, which succeed in traversing the vagina and reaching the os.

PHYSIOLOGICAL AND PSYCHOLOGICAL EFFECTS.—The effects vary according to the type of man practising the method and with the frequency of coitus and the duration of the habit. Absolute condemnation of the method is not unanimous. Kenneth Walker says that, "although there are many examples of harm inflicted by it, there are still more numerous cases in which it has apparently resulted neither in sexual weakness nor neurosis."—("Male Disorders of Sex," p. 112.)

In France, inquiries on behalf of the National Committee of Maternal Health of America revealed that a substantial majority of medical men, gynæcologists and neurologists believed the method to be probably harmless.

Dr. Abraham Stone, speaking at the International Birth Control Conference at Zurich, 1930, said :—

> " I have seen a number of men who had continued coitus interruptus for many years without any apparent ill-effects, either organic or functional. The prostate remained normal in size and consistency, the prostatic secretion was normal in cellular content, and the posterior urethra showed no evidence of congestion or of enlargement of the veru through the posterior endoscope."

It is, however, generally agreed that the following harmful effects may result from the practice of withdrawal over a period in certain cases :—

A. *On the Male*

1. Persistent hyperæmia in the lumbar centres and in the sex organs, leading to (*a*) changes in the prostate and the posterior urethra ; and (*b*) hyper-irritability and final exhaustion of the nerve centres, with consequent partial or complete impotence.
2. Psycho-neurotic manifestations (*e.g.*, anxiety neurosis) due to the tension of watchfulness so as to time withdrawal and to the effort necessary to effect this at a time when there should be complete abandon.

B. *On the Female*

1. If the act is not carried to its natural conclusion by orgasm achieved after withdrawal, delayed detumescence leads to chronic congestion of the pelvic organs, associated with such symptoms as backache, menorrhagia and painful ovary.
2. Anxiety, for fear of failure to time withdrawal successfully, leads to inhibition of normal sex response, which in some cases causes complete frigidity and active dislike of the sexual act.
3. The mental effect of repeated frustration causes psychic trauma resulting in psycho-neurosis, with such symptoms as insomnia, irritability and emotional instability.

The effects on the female are again very variable, and depend to a great extent upon :—

(*a*) Whether she is sexually aroused or not.

(*b*) Whether she experiences orgasm, either before or after withdrawal.

In the modification of this method—coitus prolongatus—withdrawal is postponed until *after* the female orgasm has occurred, and the woman consequently suffers comparatively little or no ill-effect.

I have little doubt that a considerable number of married women—particularly among the worried and under-nourished mothers of the clinic class—submit to coitus without themselves experiencing any sexual excitement or satisfaction, irrespective of the adoption of any birth control methods. These women appear to suffer no ill-effects from coitus interruptus, apart from fear of failure, and have no personal objection to it until experience shows its unreliability.

Coitus interruptus, in common with the condom method of contraception, deprives the woman of the seminal fluid. The question of the beneficial absorption of elements of the semen is still regarded as unsettled, but it must be kept in mind as a possible further objection to the method of withdrawal.

The advantages of coitus interruptus—convenience, cheapness and accessibility—are obvious.

Its disadvantages are unreliability and possible physical and psychic injury.

Coitus Reservatus (Male Continence, Karessa, Zugassent)

Coitus reservatus is the prolongation of coitus without active movements or seminal emission. The woman may have one or more orgasms, or she also may forego orgasm entirely. Intromission is prolonged considerably. According to Stopes,

> " The union is protracted, and the erection, after being active for a length of time varying from twenty minutes to ten hours, naturally subsides before withdrawal from the vagina."—(" Contraception," p. 88.)

Van de Velde states :—

> " It has been stated that the phallus remains for over an hour within the vagina, but it is more often a matter of minutes."—(" Fertility and Sterility in Marriage," p. 294.)

EFFECTS.—In normal coitus the hyperæmia of the lumbar centres and of the sex organs disappears after ejaculation, and the deplethorised tissues revert to the resting stage during which normal recuperation takes place. Coitus without orgasm, in common with coitus interruptus, if repeated over a long period, is said to result in :—

(*a*) Organic changes in the prostate and posterior urethra.
(*b*) Hyper-irritability and subsequent exhaustion of the sex centres.
(*c*) Neurotic manifestations.

There are, however, clinical records which seem to prove that these ill-effects do not invariably occur. Coitus reservatus was practised as a method of contraception by the Oneida Community in America over a period of thirty years, coitus averaging every second or third night for two to three hours ; yet, according to Dickinson, no apparent harm was revealed by competent medical and gynæcological examination. The health and eugenic record of this Community was excellent.

RELIABILITY.—Failures are recorded, possibly due to failure of the technique, leakage of semen, or to the presence of spermatozoa in the male pre-ejaculatory secretion.

Cooper urges the use of a chemical precaution in case of seminal leakage.—(" Technique of Contraception," 1928.)

Coitus Saxonus

Coitus saxonus is the prevention of the emission of seminal fluid by pressure on the urethra at the root of the penis. During orgasm the block in the urethra forces the semen into the bladder, from which it subsequently escapes during micturition.

Coitus with Incomplete Penetration

Other things being equal, there is less likelihood of conception if the ejaculate is not deposited in the region of the os and if it drains away freely. Special coital attitudes are adopted—usually as a method complementary to the use of chemical spermicide or of a douche.

The most effective attitudes for anatomical contraception are :—

1. The sedentary attitude face to face.
2. Coitus *a tergo*, ventral or horizontal attitude.

Incomplete penetration is favoured by the axial divergence of vagina and phallus, and the free drainage of the semen is facilitated.

Reliance cannot be placed upon these modifications of the coital position for contraceptive purposes.

Lactation

There is abundant clinical evidence that ovulation and conception can occur during lactation. Records are common of conception occurring even within two or three months of delivery in spite of regular breast feeding. Ovulation may be resumed without the resumption of menstruation, so that lactation as a contraceptive method is completely unreliable.

The Safe Period

Conceptions have occurred at every stage of the menstrual cycle. One cannot predict that, in any particular case, any period in the menstrual cycle will be absolutely sterile. Women with a regular twenty-eight-day menstrual cycle are least likely to conceive during the ten days preceding menstruation, and some patients of low fertility may find that they can rely upon this *relatively* safe period (see Chapter II.).

Heat to the Testes

It is known that, in the case of certain animals, immersion of the scrotum in hot water can cause a temporary sterility without any diminution of sex responses. A rise in temperature of the scrotum arrests manufacture of spermatozoa without affecting the mature spermatozoa in storage. The onset of the sterility is, therefore, delayed until the storage reservoirs have been emptied.

The possibility of achieving a revocable sterility in men is now being investigated in America ("Control of Conception," p. 117). If we can assume that heat will have similar effects in man, the contraceptive value of this method will still depend upon the possibility of determining the duration of the preliminary fertile period and of the period of sterility; and also upon the possibility of being able to guarantee full recovery of spermatogenetic function with normal fertility.

Application of X-rays to the Ovaries

Irradiation of the ovaries is used to produce an artificial menopause, but its use and value for contraceptive purposes to produce a temporary sterility is problematical for the following reasons:—

1. We cannot at present control the dosage with sufficient accuracy to regulate with certainty the degree and duration of the sterility.
2. Women may vary in their reactions, so that an exposure which in one woman produces the desired temporary sterility may in another so damage the ovaries as to arrest ovulation permanently.
3. The possibility of genetic mutations arising from damaged ova. Such effects have been demonstrated in fruit flies and other insects.

There is no record of an increase of defective children born from women who conceived *after* the irradiation, but X-ray treatment *during* pregnancy undoubtedly results in a large proportion of defective offspring.

Dr. Sv. Stefanik (Bratislavské Lekárske Listy, February, 1933) records the results of the application of X-rays to the ovaries in order to produce temporary sterilisation in 103 cases. In 12·1 per cent. the treatment was unsuccessful, and in 6·8 per cent. of these cases permanent sterility resulted. He recommends the method of temporary X-ray sterilisation in exceptional cases only.

CHAPTER IX

CONTRACEPTION FOR THE NORMAL WOMAN

General Considerations

Æsthetic Difficulties.—It is idle to overlook or to disregard the fact that any method of conception control which depends upon the use of chemicals or upon the manipulation of appliances by husband or wife, or which interferes with the natural spontaneity of intercourse, is distasteful to many people, and may seriously lessen or destroy sexual satisfaction.

That this distaste has its origin in sex inhibitions is quite immaterial to the patient. The distaste *does* exist, it may be unconquerable, and its effects may be serious. People of a scientific type of mind are apt to overlook that, to many women, a gynæcological examination alone is a terrifying and distressing experience. Many patients enter my consulting room nervous and embarrassed, and confess that it has taken them some months to raise the courage to come for advice on birth control, and that only dire necessity has finally brought them. It is well worth while to spend time in tactful and sympathetic reassurance before taking the medical history. In birth control work, perhaps more than in any other, we need constantly to keep in mind that we are dealing with human beings whose outlook necessarily differs from that of the scientist. There are patients who are nauseated by any manipulations of the genital region, such as are necessary in douching, or in the use of an occlusive pessary, or even in the insertion of a suppository; and in some cases the husband is willing to use a condom, although he dislikes it, rather than submit his wife to a distasteful procedure. It may happen that in time the wife overcomes her sensitiveness; on the other hand, persistence in the use of a method which is distasteful may lead to increasing distaste for the sexual relationship, and ultimately to frigidity.

Convenience and Economic Considerations.—A woman who has ample leisure, facilities for obtaining hot water, and the privacy of a bathroom, has a wider choice of acceptable contraceptive methods than a typical clinic patient of the poorest class, living with husband and several children in one room, and possibly sharing a lavatory with several other families in conditions of extreme poverty. In such circumstances the patient will very likely abandon in despair a method which involves frequently repeated expenditure, or demands the privacy necessary for douching, or in fact any elaborate technique.

A method which is suitable during the normal home life may have to be modified during holidays or travel. In short, not only should the economic social conditions be kept in mind when selecting a method, but, in addition, a patient should be advised that other methods are available for special circumstances, or whenever the particular method she is using proves inconvenient for any reason.

The Personal Factor.—Even the most effective of the generally accepted present-day methods of contraception will fail unless the patient has the ability and intelligence to carry out properly the instructions given. Apart from questions of convenience and expense, the intelligence of the patient is a factor which must govern the choice of a method. For mental defectives and patients of low-grade mentality the ideal would be some method of achieving a revocable or permanent sterility which does not depend upon the patient's forethought and intelligence, but is completely controlled by the doctor. Such independence of the patient's co-operation on each occasion of coitus is the theoretical advantage of biological methods and of the intra-uterine rings.

Apart from the condom—which is in some cases unacceptable to the husband—*the consensus of opinion among medical men and women who are most experienced in birth control work is that, at present, an occlusive pessary combined with a chemical contraceptive or douche gives the best results.* Our clinic patients include women sent from mental hospitals; but in our experience, provided the necessary time can be given to teaching, it is most unusual for a patient to prove incapable of learning to adjust and remove a diaphragm pessary, although in exceptional cases a third or fourth visit for instruction may be necessary in addition to the routine second visit to the clinic. The patience and teaching ability of the doctor or nurse are of great importance, for, although the majority of patients succeed in adjusting the pessary correctly within five or ten minutes, others—by no means limited to clinic patients—need much more encouragement and help before they achieve a confident success. Except in those malpositions of the uterus which bring the axis of the cervix into line with the vaginal axis, I do not advise any attempt to instruct a mentally defective patient in the use of a cervical pessary, which is considerably more difficult to adjust and to remove than a diaphragm pessary.

Konikow states :—

> " I have fitted about five thousand women with pessaries, and have found very few unable to learn the technique easily. I even remember one patient sent me by a psychiatrist with a statement giving her mental age as eight years. She responded to instruction readily, and has found no difficulty in using the pessary." —(" Physicians Manual of Birth Control," p. 96.)

Stone, the Medical Director of the Clinical Research Bureau of New York, states :—

> " As a rule, the patient can be taught the use of the (diaphragm) pessary within five to ten minutes. There are some women, however, who find much greater difficulty in acquiring the technique. Some find it hard to grasp the elementary principles of their anatomy; others are so sexually inhibited that it takes some time to overcome their reluctance and even repugnance to touching their genitalia. The physician must exercise much patience in such instances, and, if necessary, the patient should be given the pessary to practise with at home, and she is to return for a check-up before she actually begins to use it for contraceptive purposes. In

our clinic we make it a routine to have every patient return within a week for such a check-up.

" Occasionally one encounters a patient whose mentality is so low that she cannot possibly learn the simple technique of using the pessary. The number of such women is very small. It may be interesting to note in this connection that a number of women have been referred to the Maternal Health Centre in Newark, New Jersey, by the psychiatric institutes of that State. Many of these women were suffering from feeble-mindedness or psychoses of one kind or another. Yet little difficulty has been experienced by the staff in instructing them, and the results have been very gratifying."—(" The Practice of Contraception," p. 8.)

A few patients, however, even though they succeed in learning to adjust and remove the occlusive pessary correctly, yet find the method unacceptable because they lack confidence in their ability to continue using it successfully.

The Normal Woman

I should like again to emphasise the pelvic variations in the normal healthy woman : the difference in size and shape and direction of the vagina, in the tone of the vaginal muscles, and in the size and shape of the cervix. In some patients there is no retro-pubic space, and this condition precludes the use of a diaphragm pessary in the oblique position. In other cases a small cervix in a relatively long vagina is out of reach of the patient's finger. It is by no means uncommon in multiparæ to find the upper vagina very much ballooned, so that the cervix projects freely into a relatively large cavity, and in these cases a cervical or vault pessary is the more likely to become displaced, especially during coitus, when it may be pushed up into the posterior or lateral fornix.

The nullipara, after the hymen has been sufficiently stretched or ruptured and any lacerations due to the consummation of the marriage have healed, can usually be fitted with a small size (45 to 65) diaphragm pessary (Dutch or Ramses) or a small vault pessary (Dumas or Prencap), which is lubricated with a non-greasy spermicidal ointment or jelly (see Chapter IV.). In addition, she uses either a suppository or a foam tablet or jelly, which is inserted, below the occlusive pessary, about five minutes before coitus; or, as an alternative to the use of one of these, she douches the following morning with at least a quart of liquid, removing the pessary midway in the douching process, so that the vagina is cleansed of all traces of seminal fluid before the cervix is uncovered. The second portion of the douching liquid is then used for a final irrigation of the vagina and cervix.

An alternative method is a combination of condom and chemical spermicide (suppository, tablet or jelly). Where the wife finds the manipulations involved in the use of an occlusive pessary seriously distasteful, or where the husband suffers from premature ejaculation, the condom is the method of choice.

If both the condom and the occlusive pessary are for any reason unsuitable, the spermicidal jelly, such as Mil-San, is probably the most reliable alternative.

The multipara can use the same methods, but requires usually a larger-sized pessary (diaphragm, 70 to 85, or a vault pessary, medium or large size).

In either case, where the retro-pubic space is absent, a diaphragm pessary cannot be used satisfactorily, except when it is used as a vault pessary in the alternative method of fitting; in the oblique fitting the absence of support for the anterior rim would cause the pessary to slip down in front. In such cases, therefore, the choice of pessary lies between a small-sized Dutch or Ramses, used as a vault pessary, or a Dumas, Prencap, Racial or similar type. The use of the condom and chemical spermicide is an alternative method which may be preferred by the patient and acceptable to the husband.

If any patient wishes to use a chemical method alone, she has the choice of numerous suppositories, jellies (foaming and non-foaming) and foam tablets; but in discussing alternative methods, the possibility and significance of direct ejaculation of semen on the region of the cervical os, or even into the cervical canal, and of the ineffective distribution of the spermicide should be pointed out to her, so that she may appreciate the risk of dispensing with the rubber mechanical barrier.

Special Circumstances

It is well to inform patients that methods can be changed to suit special circumstances.

The Virgin.—In those cases where an intact hymen would prevent the insertion of an occlusive pessary, the condom, well lubricated, is the method of choice. For further security a chemical spermicide can be used in addition to the condom. If the condom is unacceptable, the small nozzle used for the application of Mil-San and other spermicidal jellies can usually be inserted through the virgin introitus without difficulty. Patients should be warned not to use a foaming tablet until any lacerations due to the consummation of the marriage have healed ; otherwise, intense smarting may be caused. After about a month an occlusive pessary can be substituted for the condom if the patient prefers this. The probability of needing a larger size of pessary at the end of three or four months should be kept in mind, and the patient should be asked to return for examination after a suitable interval.

Only in those cases where the hymen has been stretched or surgically removed, or where it is so slightly developed as to offer no obstruction to the use of a small diaphragm or vault pessary, may the virgin be fitted and instructed in the use of an occlusive pessary in preparation for her marriage.

Contraception after Recent Parturition.—After childbirth, until the stretched vaginal tissues have resumed their normal tone, the patient will probably need, temporarily or permanently, a larger-sized diaphragm pessary than she used before the recent pregnancy ; or a previously used vault or cervical pessary may now be contra-indicated by the cervical lacerations resulting from the recent parturition. I advise the use of the condom for two or three months following parturition, after which, when the parts have become normal, the patient may be refitted with a diaphragm or vault pessary if she so desires. If the patient prefers to resume the use of a diaphragm pessary after her confinement, she should be refitted after the confinement, and a further examination should be made within three to six months, in case changes in the pelvic condition indicate a change in the size or type of pessary. I do not advise the fitting of an occlusive pessary until at least six weeks after the confinement.

The *soft* brown rubber Dumas pessary (Lambert's Pro-race), and the "Prencap" Dumas (Prentif Ltd.), are useful in cases of post-parturition tenderness, when the husband is unwilling or unable to use a condom.

Contraception at the Menopause.—Knowledge of the fact that pregnancy may occur at the menopause, even after menstruation has become irregular and scanty or even has ceased entirely for a few months, is responsible for the anxiety of many patients to practise some form of contraception during this time. Although the pelvic condition and the previous marital history may lead one to the opinion that the chances of pregnancy are very remote, it is sometimes advisable, for the patient's peace of mind, to instruct her in some method of contraception. In such cases it is probably justifiable to rely entirely upon a chemical method alone, unless the husband is willing to use a condom; or the patient may feel more secure if she uses an occlusive pessary. It may be wisdom to countenance—or even to recommend—more elaborate contraceptive precautions than those actually indicated in the particular case in order to allay an intense mental anxiety. The known fact that a neighbour or friend became pregnant at "the change," after perhaps an interval of several years, bears more weight than the doctor's assurance that contraception in her case is probably unnecessary, or that a chemical method alone will suffice!

Where there is no evidence of any lessening fertility, the usual combination of mechanical and chemical method should be advised. It is well to warn the patient to report any irregular or profuse hæmorrhages or any abnormal discharge at this period.

Contraception in Tropical Climates.—Ordinary rubber appliances tend to perish quickly in hot climates, especially where the humidity is high. Both rubber pessaries and condoms can be preserved by a coating of glycerine, and some firms pack both pessaries and condoms in glycerine for export to the tropics.

The writer recommends that rubber pessaries and washable sheaths should be kept *immersed* in French chalk. A diaphragm pessary preserved in this way was in regular use for four years by a patient in Ceylon, and was in a good state of preservation when brought for inspection. It is important that the rubber should be *thoroughly dried* before being stored in the French chalk. The appliance should be kept in as cool a place as possible and should not be exposed to light.

Pessaries and condoms made from latex rubber which has been cured and sterilised in boiling water only, and which is therefore free from chemical adulterants, are believed to withstand high temperatures better than the ordinary gasoline rubber. Among the chemical contraceptives, cocoa-butter intended for export to the tropics is sometimes adulterated in order to raise the melting point, and this adulteration detracts from its effectiveness as a vehicle, since not infrequently it fails to melt at body temperature. Some suppositories are encased in tin foil. The foam tablets are said to keep well in the tropics provided that they are kept airtight; they should be kept in as cool a place as possible and not exposed to bright sunlight. The foaming jelly " PermFoam " is another suitable chemical preparation for hot climates, since laboratory tests have shown that it is unaffected by a wide range of temperature.

Contraception when Travelling.—During a prolonged journey such as a sea voyage, any method of contraception which involved cleansing and sterilisation of appliances or the preparation of a douche would obviously be unsuitable. A patient may need fitting and instruction in the use of an occlusive pessary for subsequent use, but for use during the journey the condom and a chemical spermicide, or a jelly, suppository or foam tablet alone, if the condom be unacceptable, may be preferred. Jellies are packed with separate tubes and nozzles for each application, so that no cleansing and sterilisation of appliances are required.

CHAPTER X

CONTRACEPTION FOR THE ABNORMAL WOMAN

[It is assumed, of course, that any necessary treatment of the local condition will be arranged.]

The following pathological conditions are commonly met with :—

Local :

Uterine displacements of varying degrees,
prolapse,
retroversion,
acute ante-flexion,
lateral displacements.

Unhealthy cervix—laceration, erosion, ulceration.

Vaginal abnormalities, including cystocele, rectocele, adhesions, vaginal tumours and mild degrees of vaginismus.

Abnormal vaginal and cervical secretions (leucorrhœa and purulent discharges), or an abnormal dryness of the vagina.

Constipation.

General :

Mental deficiency.

Obesity.

Circulatory, respiratory, renal and other conditions which are medical indications for the avoidance of pregnancy.

Introductory.—I must repeat that there is no *completely* reliable method of contraception. Not infrequently, both in private practice and at birth control clinics, one meets with patients for whom a completely reliable method of contraception is of vital importance—to whom a pregnancy involves inevitable serious damage to health and even risk to life ; and these are the cases which are often most difficult to deal with satisfactorily. This is the most discouraging aspect of practical birth control work, and those who are familiar with these difficulties will appreciate how urgent is the need for a harmless and completely reliable method of preventing pregnancy. In my opinion, sterilisation is at present the only completely satisfactory treatment of such cases; and, according to the publication of the Committee for Legalising Eugenic Sterilisation, voluntary *therapeutic* sterilisation is legal. They state (p. 14):—

> "As to the legality of sterilising a person in the interest of his *own* health (*i.e.*, for therapeutic reasons), there is no ambiguity. Such an operation is unquestionably legal, and is frequently performed. Women are often sterilised if conception would prove dangerous to life, and men when it is imperative on medical grounds."

Unfortunately, the opportunities for therapeutic sterilisation are quite inadequate to meet the need, and we have to advise the best contraceptive measures in the circumstances, knowing full well that complete protection against pregnancy cannot be guaranteed.

Another group of cases includes those patients, usually the mothers of large families living in conditions of bad housing and poverty, who for humane reasons should not be subjected to the strain of further pregnancies, although one cannot maintain that further pregnancy would be dangerous to life. The legal position in regard to the voluntary sterilisation of such patients appears to be somewhat ambiguous, but the general opinion is that sterilisation for such reasons is illegal. It is common knowledge, however, that sterilising operations are not infrequently performed in the course of abdominal operations, such as Cæsarian section, appendicectomy, etc. The patient or her husband could, in the present state of the law, bring an action for damages against the doctor at some future time. It is difficult to imagine, however, that any jury would award more than purely nominal damages in such a case. Nevertheless, I think that voluntary sterilisation for medical reasons which do not involve danger to life, with proper safeguards, should be made legal; as at present it is the only *absolutely* reliable method of preventing pregnancy.

Local Conditions

Uterine Prolapse.—Whether or not an occlusive rubber pessary can be used depends upon the degree of the prolapse and the tone of the vaginal walls. Where a uterine support is used, usually an occlusive pessary cannot be adjusted satisfactorily, and the condom or the sponge, together with a chemical spermicide, should be suggested as an alternative. In some cases of uterine prolapse it is possible to use a diaphragm pessary satisfactorily, provided there is sufficient tone in the vaginal walls and a deep retro-pubic space for the adequate support of the rim. Cervical or vault pessaries are generally less reliable than a diaphragm where there is even a moderate degree of uterine prolapse, because, *inter alia*, of the greater liability to displacement; there is considerable range of passive movement of the uterus during coitus. The final choice will rest upon actual clinical trial, and the patient should be urged to report any discomfort or displacement of the pessary. In many such cases the condom proves to be the most suitable method; but, unfortunately, the condom does not always prove acceptable to the husband.

Cystocele and Rectocele.—The presence of a cystocele means, usually, that the retro-pubic space is obliterated and consequently there is no support for the anterior rim of a Dutch or Ramses diaphragm pessary. The choice of a pessary in such a case lies between a Matrisalus diaphragm, a small fitting Dutch or Ramses used as a vault pessary, or a Dumas, Prencap, Pro-race or Racial. My own experience of fitting the Matrisalus diaphragm in such cases has not been entirely satisfactory, but it may prove useful in special cases. If none of these proves satisfactory, the condom, lubricated with spermicidal jelly, or the sponge or tampon, together with an effective chemical agent (suppository, foaming tablet, jelly, medicated douche, etc.), must be considered.

A cystocele which develops immediately after a confinement may present only temporary difficulties, as the condition not uncommonly clears up with the general restoration of muscle tone. I have seen such cases become quite normal within three months of labour with adequate post-natal care, including graduated exercises. Re-examination after this interval may therefore reveal that a return to the use of a Dutch or Ramses diaphragm pessary is possible.

The rectocele of itself does not necessarily interfere with the fitting of the posterior rim of a diaphragm pessary, unless it is associated with a loaded rectum. When the rectum is empty, the posterior rim of the diaphragm slides over the bulging recto-vaginal septum into the posterior fornix, provided that pressure is applied in the right direction, although the difficulties of insertion are naturally increased. However, the use of the diaphragm pessary in cases of rectocele is usually contra-indicated on account of the associated constipation and the co-existent cystocele.

The same limitations and precautions apply here as in the case of cystocele.

A uniform laxity of vaginal tissue with excessive secretions would be an indication for an alum douche or other astringent as part of the contraceptive technique.

Acute Retroversion, Ante-flexion or Lateral Displacements.—In my opinion, the diaphragm pessary is suitable for the majority of such cases provided a satisfactory fit can be obtained between the rim of the pessary and the vaginal wall. The exact position of the cervix is immaterial so long as it is covered by the loose rubber diaphragm and can be felt through the rubber by the patient. It is sometimes more difficult to teach the patient to identify her cervix in the first place, but, provided this difficulty can be overcome, I have found that the diaphragm pessary is perfectly satisfactory in many such cases.

In acute ante-flexion and retroversion the axis of the cervix is brought into line, more or less, with the vaginal axis. A vault pessary in such cases is less likely to be displaced by the movements of the phallus than when the uterus is in the normal position. On this account, and because they believe that there is a likelihood of exposure of the cervix between the rim of a diaphragm pessary and the vaginal wall in such displacements, Konikow and others recommend the vault pessary for cases of retroversion and acute ante-flexion. I prefer the diaphragm pessary when possible, provided that the patient can be taught to slide the rim of the diaphragm *behind* the cervix into the posterior fornix. I have rarely found, in these displacements, that the entering rim is more liable to slide up in front of the cervix than in normal cases. Whenever this exposure of the cervix occurs, it is due to failure to adopt and maintain the right direction of that part of the pessary which first enters the vagina—failure to slide the rim along without losing contact with the posterior vaginal wall until it reaches the posterior fornix. (See instructions for using a diaphragm pessary, p. 83 (*e*).)

Lacerations, Erosions and other Pathological Conditions of the Cervix.—The leucorrhœa, which is associated with cervical catarrh and cervical erosion, constitutes a common difficulty in birth control work, especially among multiparæ. It is obviously desirable that the secretion should not be held up for any length of time in the vagina; and where a diaphragm pessary is used in cases with a profuse discharge, it is best to advise the removal of the pessary and the administration of a medicated douche, such as the "G.P." douche or lactic acid (1 drachm to the quart), within about an hour of coitus. Such a modification of the usual procedure robs it of the advantage of needing no disturbance or manipulation until the following morning. On this account the patient may well prefer the condom; or to take the possibly greater risk of pregnancy by relying upon a jelly, suppository or foam tablet alone, and postponing the douche until the following morning.

It should always be kept in mind that local injuries and infection due to child-birth, including cervicitis and cervical laceration, are "important predisposing causes of cancer of the cervix" (p. 126, "Final Report of Departmental Committee on Maternal Mortality and Morbidity," Ministry of Health, 1932). It is obviously important to avoid, as far as possible, anything which causes or may cause chronic irritation in such cases, and for this reason I regard the condom as the method of choice where it is acceptable; or, as an alternative, a diaphragm which, if there is a profuse discharge, is removed shortly after coitus, with the usual additional precautions. *Cervical caps are definitely contra-indicated.* A spermicide which is also a germicide, such as PermFoam jelly, Mil-San jelly, Antipart tablets and Prensols, is especially useful in such cases.

Constipation.—Patients should be warned that constipation may cause the fitting of a diaphragm pessary to be so defective as to render it ineffectual. A distended rectum causes irregular bulging of the posterior vaginal wall, and this prevents a sufficiently close and uniform contact with the rim of the pessary. Such a condition is readily perceptible to the patient when she is attempting to insert the pessary—an operation which is rendered much more difficult by the distortion of the vaginal cavity—and she should not attempt to use the pessary until the lower bowel has been emptied. In cases of chronic constipation, therefore, it is usually advisable to substitute for the diaphragm pessary a vault pessary or a condom, at any rate until the constipation has been corrected.

Vaginal Spasm.—A mild degree of vaginismus is sometimes encountered which, although not preventing coitus, causes dyspareunia, and prevents the use of an occlusive pessary. In such cases one can advise a well-lubricated condom, or a foaming tablet or jelly, or a suppository, until the condition is overcome. Of course, any local lesion, such as a tender caruncle, should be treated.

General Conditions

Mental Deficiency.—The mentally defective patient may prove unteachable; and even if she be capable of learning to adjust and remove an occlusive pessary, the probability is that she will fail to carry out the method consistently, and so will fail to avoid undesirable pregnancies.

The husband may be willing and capable of using a condom properly lubricated with a contraceptive jelly, and if this method can be combined with the use of a chemical contraceptive by the wife a high degree of security against conception will be attained.

For complete protection against pregnancy, sterilisation is necessary; *no method of contraception is absolutely reliable.*

METHODS OF STERILISATION.—In the male—vasectomy.

In the female :—

(*a*) Salpingectomy.

(*b*) Intra-uterine cauterisation of the uterine ends of the Fallopian tubes.

(*c*) Production of artificial menopause by application of X-rays to the ovaries.

Other methods of sterilisation, *still in the experimental stage*, include :—

(*d*) Injection of sperms, to act as immunising vaccines forming antibodies.

(*e*) Injection of extracts of corpus luteum, which prevent the development of the Graafian follicles and suppress menstruation.

(*f*) Injections of folliculin, or insulin, or of extract of the anterior lobe of the pituitary.

(*g*) Diet deficient in vitamin E.

PRESENT LEGAL POSITION REGARDING STERILISATION.—*Voluntary therapeutic sterilisation* is the only form of sterilisation which can be legally performed.

The British Medical Association obtained counsel's opinion regarding the legal aspect of the sterilisation of *mental defectives who are too defective to be able to give their consent.* Sir Travers Humphreys stated (*Brit. Med. Journ.*, June, 1925, p. 286) :—

> " I am clearly of opinion that any medical man who performs the operation described upon a 'defective' within the meaning of that term as defined within the Mental Deficiency Act, 1913, would in the present state of law be acting illegally and without any legal justification. I assume the consent of both parents and the excellence of the motives of all concerned, but the fact remains that the operation of sterilisation involves an

assault upon and the wounding of the person operated upon. The only legal justification for such an action in regard to a person who either from extreme youth or old age or from any other cause such as mental weakness, is incapable of giving a reasoned consent, would be that the operation was necessary to the health or well-being of the patient.

"The legal risks involved in such an operation would attach equally to all the persons concerned—that is the doctor who performs it, and the parent or guardian who requested or sanctioned it. . . ."

In regard to the *voluntary sterilisation* of mentally deficients or of any other persons, Lord Riddell (*loc. cit.*, p. 5) expresses the view that voluntary sterilisation, no less than that undertaken when the patient is incapable of giving his consent, is illegal. This view is based on obsolete legislation concerned with the prohibition against maiming.

Obesity.—Marked obesity may make it extremely difficult or even impossible for a patient to adjust or remove an occlusive pessary, especially a pessary of the vault or cervical type. Relatively short fingers or a long vagina increase the difficulty. Even if she succeed in putting the pessary into the vagina, the patient may be quite unable (unless the uterus is so low, either through prolapse or through shortness of the vagina, as to bring the cervix well within reach of her finger) to confirm the correct placing of the pessary by feeling the cervix through the soft rubber dome of a diaphragm, Prencap, soft brown rubber Dumas or cervical cap, or over the rim of the thicker white rubber Dumas.

In these cases, if the diaphragm (Dutch or Ramses) prove unsuitable, the condom should next be considered as an alternative; but if the condom prove unacceptable, the patient may try a thin, flat rubber sponge, cut specially if necessary, to cover adequately her vaginal vault and fitted, where necessary, with a tag to facilitate removal, and soaked in a spermicidal solution, such as vinegar and water; or a medicated tampon of cotton-wool, to be destroyed after use, may be used. In any case, the use of a tampon or sponge should be combined with the additional protection of a jelly, suppository or foam tablet inserted below the tampon, or a douche taken the following morning, the sponge or tampon being removed midway in the douching process.

Some patients, however, find that the bulk of sponge or wool required to cover adequately the vaginal vault causes definite discomfort during coitus. Reliance must then be placed, as a last resource, on a chemical spermicide alone, such as a foaming or non-foaming jelly, a foaming tablet, or a suppository. Mil-San, PermFoam, Antipart, Semori or large Prensols may be advised. Rendell's suppositories are relatively efficient spermicides but contain quinine (see p. 46). The selection is limited by the economic condition of the patient. One must recognise, however, that the absence of a mechanical barrier over the cervix constitutes a certain amount of risk of failure.

Chronic Diseases of the Heart, Lungs, Kidneys, Nervous System, etc.—In cases where pregnancy would be detrimental to health, aggravating existing disease or even causing risk to life, the responsibility of giving contraceptive advice is a very grave one. Where possible it is advisable to recommend a combination of occlusive pessary, chemical spermicide and douche—as, for example, a Dutch pessary lubricated with G.P. ointment and Mil-San or Prensols or Antipart inserted before coitus and a douche the following morning—or a condom and chemical spermicide, with additional measures (see p. 104) after coitus should the condom tear. However, economic difficulties may prohibit the use of the most effective chemical spermicides, and the patient may be unable to be fitted satisfactorily with any kind of occlusive pessary, and the husband may refuse or be unable to use a condom; even a sponge or tampon may be unsuitable for local reasons. For such cases voluntary sterilisation for husband or wife should be available.

CHAPTER XI

EVALUATION OF CONTRACEPTIVE METHODS

IN comparing statistics of the results of methods of contraception, difficulties arise owing to the lack of common standards of assessment and lack of uniformity in the use of terminology.

The differences in the interpretation of the term " failure " illustrate this difficulty. Florence (" Birth Control on Trial," p. 71), referring to her analysis of the results of the first 300 cases of the Cambridge Clinic, states :—

> " We feel that a contraceptive can be legitimately classed as a success only when it has actually been used with success over a considerable period of time—that is, when it has not been so difficult or painful or obnoxious that the patient had to give it up, and when it has definitely prevented conception. And we feel that, in general, the other cases must be classed as failures whether that failure occurred when the appliance was being properly used, or after it had been given up, either because the patient's condition was not sufficiently normal to permit of its use, or because the appliance caused pain, or because the patient found it so distasteful that she could not continue, or because she was too nervous and frightened to use it and had no confidence in it, or even because she was too stupid to apply it successfully."

She therefore includes as failures of the method those patients who have for various reasons abandoned the method and have then become pregnant. On the other hand, the Manchester Clinic, in their Annual Report, recognised as failures only those cases who became pregnant in spite of using correctly the full method on all occasions. The Seventh International Birth Control Conference (Zurich, 1930) recommended that the term " failure " be restricted to cases in which the patient conceives in spite of using the method prescribed. The Society for the Provision of Birth Control Clinics has adopted the following classification of unsatisfactory results :—

A. *Failure of method.*

1. Apparently used correctly.
2. Due to incomplete following of instructions.
3. Due to lapses from continuity.
4. Due to deteriorated or faulty appliance.
5. Due possibly to constipation.
6. Other causes.

B. *Unacceptability to patient of advice given.*

1. Æsthetic dislike.
2. Discomfort caused to the husband.
3. Discomfort caused to the wife.
4. The " too much trouble " type of case.
5. Other causes.

August, 1930.

WALWORTH WOMEN'S WELFARE CENTRE

Summary of First 7,000 *Patients First Attending between November*, 1921–*March*, 1927

	* Dutch and Soapy Douche.	* Dumas and Soapy Douche.	* Unique and Soapy Douche.	Sheath.	Soluble.	Total.
Successful	2,143	379	57	304	10	2,893
Failure, apparently used correctly	26	10	1	—	2	39
Failure due to inserting wrongly	7	14	—	—	—	21
Failure due to faulty appliance	21	4	1	8	—	34
Failure due to omitting to syringe	32	3	—	—	—	35
Failure due to cause unknown	40	9	2	1	—	52
Not using appliance and became pregnant † . .	146	9	2	1	—	158
Not using for various reasons ‡	64	10	1	—	—	75
Pregnancy desired . . . ceased to practise contraception .	83	9	4	1	—	97
No report received . .	2,897	621	18	53	7	3,596
Total .	5,459	1,068	86	368	19	7,000

* See Detailed Analysis *re* numbers using Ointment or Solubles in addition.

† On holiday 23
Appliance worn out and did not renew . . . 18
Lost and did not renew 8
Other causes, generally due to omission on one occasion 109

158

‡ Summary of those not using appliance for various reasons :—
Husband or wife dead 9
Dislike of method . . . . 18 (11 Dutch, 6 Dumas, 1 Unique)
Husband objects . . . . . 20 (18 Dutch, 2 Dumas)
Wearing ring 6
Lack of confidence . . . . 4 (3 Dutch, 1 Dumas)
Sterilised 6
Too much trouble . . . . 2 (Dutch)
No reason . . . . . . 5 (3 Dutch, 2 Dumas)
Prefer coitus interruptus . . . 4 (1 Dutch, 2 Dumas)
Could not manage . . . . 1 (Dutch)

75

Of the first 8,000 *cases :* 554 were pregnant on first visit.
30 sought advice for apparent sterility.

August, 1930.

Walworth Women's Welfare Centre

Analysis of the First 7,000 *Patients First Attending between November*, 1921–*March*, 1927

(*Note.*—Patients who for various reasons were not given birth control information have been eliminated.)

Successful.	Period of Report.									Total.	Grand Totals.	
	6 + mths.	1 + yr.	2+ yrs.	3+ yrs.	4+ yrs.	5+ yrs.	6+ yrs.	7+ yrs.	8+ yrs.			
1. Dutch pessary and soapy douche .	183	113	185	94	74	57	45	24	9	784		
Dutch ointment and soapy douche.	115	309	263	293	196	94	37	8	5	1,320		
Dutch soluble and soapy douche .	6	5	5	9	9	3	1	1	—	39	2,143	
2. Dumas pessary and soapy douche .	3	15	8	9	10	14	—	—	—	59		
Dumas ointment and soapy douche	27	84	47	70	47	23	2	—	—	300		
Dumas soluble and soapy douche .	2	6	1	5	4	1	1	—	—	20	379	
3. Unique and soapy douche . .	1	7	10	8	3	2	2	—	—	33		
Unique ointment and soapy douche	1	7	4	2	7	2	—	—	—	23		
Unique soluble and soapy douche .	—	1	—	—	—	—	—	—	—	1	57	
4. Sheath	4	33	87	70	48	32	11	2	—	287		
Sheath and soluble . . .	1	3	4	1	3	5	—	—	—	17	304	
5. Soluble (quinine or lactic acid) .	2	4	2	—	2	—	—	—	—	10	10	2,893
Failure or Method not Used.												
1. Dutch pessary and douche, apparently used correctly . . .	2	3	1	—	—	—	—	—	—	6		
Dutch pessary douche and ointment, apparently used correctly . .	2	5	8	4	—	—	—	—	—	19		
Dutch pessary and soluble, apparently used correctly . . .	—	—	1	—	—	—	—	—	—	1		
Dutch pessary, used incorrectly .	3	1	1	1	—	1	—	—	—	7		
Dutch pessary (faulty) . .	—	3	8	4	5	—	—	1	—	21		
Dutch pessary, but omitted to syringe	6	8	14	3	1	—	—	—	—	32		
Dutch pessary—reason not known.	6	18	11	2	3	—	—	—	—	40	126	
2. Dumas pessary, apparently used correctly	2	3	4	—	1	—	—	—	—	10		
Dumas pessary, used incorrectly .	—	10	3	1	—	—	—	—	—	14		
Dumas pessary (faulty pessary) .	—	2	1	1	—	—	—	—	—	4		
Dumas pessary, but omitted to syringe	1	—	1	—	1	—	—	—	—	3		
Dumas pessary—reason not known.	2	1	3	2	1	—	—	—	—	9	40	
3. Unique and ointment and douche, apparently used correctly . .	—	—	—	—	1	—	—	—	—	1		
Unique, etc.—(faulty pessary) .	—	—	—	—	1	—	—	—	—	1		
Unique, etc.—reason not known .	—	2	—	—	—	—	—	—	—	2	4	
4. Sheath	1	2	4	—	1	—	—	—	—	8		
Sheath—reason not known . .	—	—	1	—	—	—	—	—	—	1	9	
5. Soluble	1 (lactic acid)	—	1	(quinine)		—	—	—	—	2	2	181
Not using and became pregnant. Dutch .	9	38	44	34	11	9	1	—	—	146		
Dumas .	2	1	3	2	1	—	—	—	—	9		
Unique .	—	2	—	—	—	—	—	—	—	2		
Sheath .	—	—	1	—	—	—	—	—	—	1		158
Not using for various reasons. Dutch .	19	15	21	5	2	2	—	—	—	64		
Dumas .	3	4	3	—	—	—	—	—	—	10		
Unique .	1	—	—	—	—	—	—	—	—	1		75
Pregnancy desired . . Dutch .	—	20	33	18	9	3	—	—	—	83		
Dumas .	—	2	3	3	—	1	—	—	—	9		
Unique .	—	1	2	1	—	—	—	—	—	4		
Sheath .	—	—	1	—	—	—	—	—	—	1		97
No report received . . Dutch .										2,897		
Dumas .										621		
Unique .										18		
Sheath .										53		
Soluble .										7		3,596
												7,000

August, 1930.

EAST LONDON WOMEN'S WELFARE CENTRE

Summary of First 1,000 *Patients First Attending between June*, 1926–*June*, 1928

	* Dutch and Soapy Douche.	* Dumas and Soapy Douche.	* Unique and Soapy Douche.	Sheath.	Soluble.	Total.
Successful	331	137	3	26	—	497
Failure, apparently used correctly	5	1	—	—	—	6
Failure due to faulty appliance	1	—	—	1	—	2
Failure due to omitting to syringe	4	2	1	—	—	7
Failure due to cause unknown	3	—	—	—	—	3
Not using appliance and became pregnant . .	12	5	—	—	—	17
Not using for various reasons †	8	1	—	—	—	9
Pregnancy desired . . . ceased to practise contraception .	13	4	1	1	—	19
No report received . .	281	140	—	18	1	440
Total .	658	290	5	46	1	1,000

* See Detailed Analysis *re* numbers using Ointment or Solubles in addition.

† Summary of those not using for various reasons :—

2 Husband away.
1 Husband dead.
1 Could not manage.
1 Reason not given (Dumas).
1 Does not feel safe.
3 Husband objects.

Of the first 1,118 *cases* :—

108 were pregnant on first visit and have not returned.
10 sought advice for apparent sterility.

August, 1930.

East London Women's Welfare Centre

Analysis of the First 1,000 *Patients First Attending between June*, 1926–*June*, 1928

(*Note.*—Patients who for various reasons were not given birth control information have been eliminated.)

	Period of Report.					Total.	Grand Totals.	
	6 + mths.	1 + year.	2 + yrs.	3 + yrs.	4 + yrs.			
Successful.								
1. Dutch pessary and soapy douche	5	15	7	10	6	43		
Dutch ointment & soapy douche	32	93	87	59	13	284		
Dutch soluble and soapy douche	—	1	2	1	—	4	331	
2. Dumas pessary and soapy douche	1	3	5	1	—	10		
Dumas ointment & soapy douche	17	24	58	16	7	122		
Dumas soluble and soapy douche	—	2	2	1	—	5	137	
3. Unique and soapy douche .	—	1	1	1	—	3	3	
4. Sheath	—	7	8	3	1	19		
Sheath and soluble . . .	—	1	1	4	1	7	26	497
Failure or Ceased to Practise Contraception.								
1. Dutch, apparently used correctly	1	2	2	—	—	5		
Dutch (faulty)	—	—	—	1	—	1		
Dutch, but omitted to syringe .	—	3	—	1	—	4		
Dutch, reason not known .	1	2	—	—	—	3	13	
2. Dumas, apparently used correctly	1	—	—	—	—	1		
Dumas, but omitted to syringe .	—	1	—	1	—	2	3	
3. Unique, but omitted to syringe .	—	1	—	—	—	1	1	
4. Sheath	—	1	—	—	—	1	1	18
Not using pessary and became pregnant. Dutch .	4	3	1	3	1	12		
Dumas	2	2	—	—	1	5	17	17
Not using pessary for various reasons. Dutch .	6	1	1	—	—	8		
Dumas	1	—	—	—	—	1	9	9
Baby desired after using Dutch .	1	7	5	—	—	13		
Dumas	—	—	4	—	—	4		
Unique	—	—	—	1	—	1		
Sheath.	—	1	—	—	—	1	19	19
No report received : Dutch .	—	—	—	—	—	281		
Dumas	—	—	—	—	—	140		
Sheath.	—	—	—	—	—	18		
Soluble	—	—	—	—	—	1	440	440
								1,000

Conference of Medical Officers of Birth Control Clinics, October, 1930, affiliated to the Society for the Provision of Birth Control Clinics

Enquiry into Failures and Unacceptability Cases

Table I.—*Cases which had Maintained Contact with Clinics*

[Results of " Follow-up " Home Visits not included]

Clinics.	Totals of Cases seen.	TOTAL of FAILURES analysed into :	Unaccountable failures.	Defect failures.	Omission failures.	Insufficient Information.	Total of UNACCEPTABILITY analysed into :	Æsthetic dislike.	Discomfort to Husband.	Discomfort to Wife.	" Too much Trouble " Type.	Other causes.	Method given up and followed by unwanted pregnancy.
Walworth . .	3,404	181	39	34	56	52	212	8	11	10	19	30	134
Aberdeen . .	492	12	4	0	6	2	17	1	2	5	1	—	8
Birmingham . .	198	25	4	4	14	3	19	2	1	1	7	—	8
East London . .	560	18	6	2	7	3	22	—	3	1	—	1	17
Newcastle . .	114	7	4	0	2	1	3	—	—	—	—	I.RC	2
N. Kensington .	1,000	60	23	12	22	3	185	9	15	21	10	84	46
Oxford . . .	76	8	2	2	2	2	3	—	—	—	—	—	3
Rotherham . .	276	7	1	1	2	3	4	—	—	—	—	—	4
Totals .	6,120	318	83	55	111	69	465	20	32	38	37	116	222

Summary :
Of the 6,120 cases analysed—
318 Failures (including unaccountable, defect and omission failures)
= about 1 in 19, or about 5 per cent.
465 Method Unacceptable
= about 1 in 13, or about 7·7 per cent.

I.—Additional Statistics from North Kensington Clinic

Cases "Followed up" by Home Visits

460 cases.

Failures, 40. About 1 in 12 or about 9 per cent.

Method unacceptable, 289. About 2 in 3, or over 60 per cent.

II.—Statistics from Cambridge Clinic

The following supplementary Tables II and III and comments have been submitted by the Cambridge Clinic.

TABLE II

Summary of 500 Cases Seen at Clinic

Table.		No.	Per cent.	Mrs. Florence's cases.	Per cent.
I	Using appliances with success .	200	61·2	92	37·2
II	Using appliances every time but failing to carry out method properly or using defective appliances. *Pregnancy resulting*	22	6·7	22	9·0
III	Appliances given up. *Pregnancy resulting*	42	12·8	53	21·5
IV	Appliances given up for C.I. *No pregnancy resulting* so far, pregnancy being unwanted .	48	14·7	60	24·3
V	Appliances given up as no longer needed	15	4·6	20	8·1
	Total . .	327	—	247	—
	Using appliances less than six months	6	—	0	—
	Not given birth control advice .	96	—	28	—
	Untraceable or not yet visited .	71	—	25	—
	Total . .	500	—	300	—

Of the 327 cases about whom data are available, 155 were visited in their homes since they had not visited this clinic for six months or longer; and 162 had visited the clinic within six months of when the data about their case were compiled.

The above table (No. II) contains a tabulated comparison of the findings of Mrs. Sargent Florence, as set forth in her book, " Birth Control on Trial " (G. A. Unwin Ltd., London, 1925) and of Mrs. Ramsey, who has pursued the same investigations up till May, 1931. One hundred and fifty of Mrs. Ramsey's 500 cases entered into Mrs. Florence's earlier series. Mrs. Florence's cases were numbered 1–300; Mrs. Ramsey's 151–650 inclusive. Thus the first 150 patients who visited the clinic do not enter into Mrs. Ramsey's list.

Florence investigation—9 per cent. failures.

Ramsey investigation—6·7 per cent. failures.

TABLE III

Successful Use of Appliances

No.	Method.	Time in Use.				Total.
		3–4½ yrs.	2–2.11 yrs.	1–1.11 yrs.	6–11 mths.	
1	Sheath	26	30	38	13	107
2	Dutch pessary, with ointment, quinine and urea pellet and douching as a rule, but not always	11	12	18	9	50
3	Dutch pessary or *sheath* used alternatively . . .	8	2	8	2	20
4	Sheath and pessary used together	—	1	1	—	2
5	*Check pessaries* . . .	2	3	1	0	6
6	*Dumas pessary* . . .	2	0	1	0	3
7	Soluble pessary alone (not taught at clinic) . .	—	1	4	1	6
8	Sponge and ointment . .	—	2	—	—	2
9	S.O.S. jelly alone (not taught at clinic) . . .	—	1	—	—	1
10	Sheath or coitus interruptus (alternately) . . .	2	1	—	—	3
	Totals . .	51	53	71	25	200

By the term " successful use of appliances " is here meant that the couples advised found the method recommended successful in preventing pregnancies. It will be noted that, out of a total of 200, over half the cases quoted are using sheaths (107 are using sheaths alone and 20 are using them alternately with the Dutch pessaries). It is the view of the Cambridge Clinic that if the husband is prepared to use it, the sheath is the most reliable method, provided the printed instructions issued with the sheath are adhered to.

General Comment.—The usual combination of chemical and mechanical methods in common use by clinic and private patients in this and other countries succeeds in its immediate aim if it prevents the ingress of spermatozoa into the uterus, whether or not an ovum be present awaiting fertilisation. From the work of Walton and others on certain mammals, there is reason to think that conception is possible only during a very brief phase—possibly not more than twenty-four hours—of the menstrual cycle. In the majority of instances, therefore, the fact that pregnancy does not result is not a proof that the contraceptive method adopted has been successful in preventing a conception; sperms may have succeeded in entering the uterus on occasions when no ovum was present in the tubes. The method is put to the test only during the period of viability of the extruded ovum and of spermatozoa present within the female genital tract. Nevertheless, the presumption is that the method is succeeding if it prevents the birth of children to a healthy couple, still in the child-bearing age, whose fertility is assured by previous conceptions and whose sexual habits remain unchanged, over a period which exceeds the natural spacing of the births. We must bear in mind that subsequent disease may cause sterility. In the case of childless couples there is, of course, no indication of natural fertility. In most cases, if not in all, it is impossible to assess with perfect accuracy the degree of success of any particular contraceptive method; and for comparative purposes, the period of sterility since its adoption is the only practicable measure of its success.

It should be remembered that clinic cases include patients

of low-grade intelligence—many referred from mental hospitals—and also patients whose domestic environment and economic limitations are serious obstacles to the successful use of present methods. They include, too, a considerable proportion of patients whose pelvic abnormalities render difficult or impossible the use of any mechanical appliance by the woman, and whose husbands refuse or are unable to use a condom.

In these circumstances, bearing in mind the real difficulties of preventing conception, the clinic results are surprisingly good where the methods prove acceptable; but the writer agrees with the conclusions expressed in the "Final Report of Departmental Committee on Maternal Mortality and Morbidity" (Ministry of Health, 1931, p. 131):—

> "It should, however, be recognised that there are no entirely reliable appliances for the prevention of pregnancy, and that it is often impracticable for women in working-class homes to use approved methods in a satisfactory and effective way. Therefore, when the avoidance of pregnancy is essential on medical grounds, the question of sterilisation should be considered."

EFFECTS ON HEALTH OF CONTRACEPTIVE METHODS

Just as harm may result from the abuse or misuse of medicines, food, and clothing, so also the use of *unsuitable* methods of contraception or the *misuse* of any particular method may be harmful, either in its immediate effects or after a period of weeks or years.

One may say definitely that the combination of methods, which has stood the test of clinical trial over a prolonged period in this and other countries, is most probably harmless when used in suitable cases. One may say, further, that it is in many cases beneficial to health and happiness, since it provides the alternative to excessive child-bearing, to abstinence from sexual intercourse during marriage, and to repeated attempts—successful and unsuccessful—to procure abortion.

Excessive child-bearing is detrimental to the health of the mother; it is also a disadvantage to the children. The Census Reports of 1911 show that there is a significant rise in infant mortality where the interval between successive births is less than two and a half years.

Douglas and McKinlay,[1] reporting on the effects of parity on maternal mortality and morbidity, show that while primiparæ have an excess risk amounting to 13 per cent., the fifth and subsequent pregnancies show a mortality greater than the first, and increasing steadily with the number of pregnancies. (It has hitherto been thought that it is not until the eighth pregnancy that the risks are greater than the first.)

The conclusion is that the effect on the maternal mortality rate of a falling birth rate is therefore generally favourable rather than the reverse, although certain causes of death such as eclampsia and accidents of childbirth would be adversely affected by the increase in the relative number of primiparæ.

The authors of this Report recommend, *inter alia*, that practical instruction in contraceptive methods should be available for women for whom further pregnancies would be dangerous.

Abstinence in marriage—except in exceptional cases or for particular reasons (pregnancy, ill-health) during limited periods—is not compatible with health and happiness. Psychiatrists, neurologists and physicians are, in the main, agreed as to the ill-effects upon normal married people of abstinence from intercourse over long periods.

Lord Dawson of Penn, speaking in the House of Lords in February, 1934, of a young couple who had had two children and who could not afford others for a period of years:—

> "They will have to practise what amounts to celibacy in the married state, and I give it as my solemn medical opinion that firstly it would be impossible; secondly, that it would destroy their health; and thirdly, that

[1] "Report on Maternal Morbidity and Mortality in Scotland," by Charlotte A. Douglas, M.D., and P. L. McKinlay, M.D., 1935 (Edinburgh: H.M. Stationery Office).

> it would force on many occasions what one always tries to avoid, and that is irregularities in sex relations—I mean within the home—perversions and eccentricities."

The Departmental Committee on Maternal Mortality and Morbidity (Interim Report, 1930, p. 45) conclude that "there can be no doubt that abortion plays a serious and regrettable part in the production of puerperal sepsis, and therefore in the causation of maternal morbidity and death. . . ." Contraception is usually the only practicable alternative to repeated attempts to procure abortions.

Harmlessness of Approved Methods

My own medical experience of the use of properly selected and properly used methods of contraception convinces me that the mechanical and chemical methods advised at the clinics of the Society for the Provision of Birth Control Clinics are harmless.

Biological tests for harmfulness of chemical contraceptives are now available, and the clinical findings of the harmlessness of the chemical contraceptives in use at these clinics, and advised by the National Birth Control Association, have been confirmed by these tests. Moreover, the large majority of clinic patients undergo examination at regular intervals, and no evidence has accrued to indicate that the practice of contraception, as advised at these clinics, has increased the incidence of pelvic lesions.

Konikow writes ("Physician's Manual of Birth Control," p. 155): "As a result of experience with several thousand patients in the last thirty years, and from special investigations of 411 cases in 1929, 200 cases in 1928, and 157 cases in 1927, I have reached the same conclusions as the physicians in charge of the various clinics who use pessaries and pastes; *i.e.*, the use of pessaries and pastes is absolutely harmless."

She states further (p. 74): "Many of my patients have used pessaries for fifteen or twenty years. I have seen and examined them many times during that period, and have found no harmful consequences!"

Under healthful methods, she groups :—

1. Intravaginal pessaries (diaphragmatic and vault) alone or in combination with douche or paste or both.
2. Mild chemicals introduced into the vagina before coitus.
3. Douches (never to be used alone).
4. Condoms.

In regard to douching, she writes (p. 63) :—

> " My re-examination of hundreds of patients using douches has not shown any change in the vaginal lining or any excessive dryness."

Chapple, in a speech at the Congress of the Royal Sanitary Institute, 1932, said :—

> " In a careful study of seventy-five thousand cases in which ordinary methods of contraception have been made use of, and which were examined very carefully, in no case was any harm shown to be done to the individual."

Florence (" Birth Control on Trial," pp. 124 and 127) observes :—

> " Our doctor has never found any evidence whatever, among those whom she has re-examined, of any harmful results following the use of a contraceptive.
>
> " Erosions and inflammation of the cervix are frequently present when the patient visits the clinic, but this condition is not increased by the use of contraceptives, and is often relieved by douching."

Charles (" The Practice of Birth Control," p. 55) says of douching :—

> " Many reputable gynæcologists regard the habitual use of a vaginal syringe as detrimental to health. It is believed by them to eliminate the protective bacteria in the vagina and thus to facilitate infections such as leucorrhœa. As far as the present material is concerned, this theory is unsubstantiated. No evidence is brought forward to indicate any detrimental effect on the health of the female."

My own comment in regard to post-coital contraceptive douching is that where leucorrhœa is already present the douche is definitely beneficial. I have not personally known the use of a douche give rise to leucorrhœa or to any pathological condition. I have seen local injury from the use of unsuitable substances, such as solutions of too great a concentration of chemicals which are quite harmless in proper dilution.

Sterility.—The Walworth Clinic provides conclusive evidence that the use of approved contraceptive methods (condoms, occlusive pessaries, spermicidal jellies, ointments, suppositories or tablets, medicated douches) does not cause sterility. Of ninety-seven patients who ceased to practise birth control because they desired a child, ninety-six became pregnant. One hundred and fifty-eight patients who reported that *on one occasion* they had neglected to use the prescribed method became pregnant.

Effect on Subsequent Pregnancy and Labour.—Referring to the suggestion that remote ill-effects might arise from the use of contraceptives, the Departmental Committee (Interim Report, p. 44) state :—

> " The Committee recognise that occasional harmful results from inflammation may be set up by mechanical or chemical agents, but apart from this fact they can find no evidence that a subsequent pregnancy or puerperium is less likely to run a normal course than in other cases."

It will be noted that this observation refers to the general public, and not to the selected class who have had medical advice on contraception, either privately or at approved clinics. It therefore includes those women who practise a method recommended by a neighbour or other unqualified person, and who use unsuitable and ill-fitting appliances and harmful chemicals.

CHAPTER XII

CONTRACEPTION AND THE PUBLIC HEALTH SERVICES

Powers of Local Authorities

THE powers of Local Authorities in England and Wales to provide facilities for advice and instruction on methods of contraception have been outlined by the Ministry of Health in Memorandum 153/M.C.W., Circular 1208, and Circular 1408, which are given verbatim in the Appendix.

According to the Memorandum, Local Authorities have no power to establish birth control clinics for the unrestricted use of married women. They may use existing institutions under their control to provide facilities for giving advice on contraceptive methods to a strictly selected class of married women *in whose cases further pregnancy would be detrimental to health.* The provision of such facilities is not compulsory, but lies within the discretion of the Local Authority.

> Under the *Notification of Births (Extension) Act*, 1915, Local Authorities may exercise the powers of the Public Health Acts by providing birth control treatment for nursing mothers.
>
> Under the *Public Health Acts* Local Authorities may provide clinics for the treatment of women suffering from gynæcological and other conditions at which married women patients may be given advice on methods of birth control if pregnancy would be detrimental to health.

The selection of suitable cases rests with the medical officer of the institution. Circular 1408 states that: "What is, or is not, medically detrimental to health must be decided by the professional judgment of the registered medical practitioner in charge of the clinic." Economic hardship alone does not provide sufficient grounds for the eligibility of a patient for contraceptive advice ; but indirectly, economic hardship, resulting from bad housing, poor nutrition and overwork, frequently leads to such impairment of health that there can be no hesitation in deciding that any further pregnancy would be detrimental to health or that definite spacing of future pregnancies is desirable on health grounds.

> In a series of 3,805 maternal deaths investigated by the Departmental Committee on Maternal Mortality and Morbidity (Final Report, 1930), 514 (13·5 per cent.) were due to lung disease, heart disease, chronic renal disease and pulmonary tuberculosis—diseases definitely made worse by pregnancy.

The Final Report of the Committee on Maternal Mortality and Morbidity, Ministry of Health, 1932, states :—

> " The Committee desire . . . to call special attention to the importance of the avoidance of pregnancy by women suffering from organic disease such as tuberculosis, heart disease, diabetes, chronic nephritis, etc., in which childbearing is likely seriously to endanger life. They consider that advice and instruction in contraceptive methods should be readily available for such women, and their husbands, from private practitioners at hospitals or at gynæcological clinics set up by Local Authorities under the Public Health Acts in accordance with suggestions made by the Ministry of Health in Circular 1208 (1931)."

The facilities that may be provided for birth control advice and instruction for the specially selected class of patient defined in the Ministry's Memorandum may be summarised as follows :—

Local Authorities

1. May establish separate birth control sessions to be held at the Maternity and Child Welfare Centres.
2. May establish birth control clinics to be held at premises separate from the Maternity and Child Welfare Centres.
3. May establish gynæcological clinics at which birth control advice may be given.

4. May refer patients to voluntary birth control clinics, the Local Authority paying a fee to be agreed upon by themselves and the clinic concerned.

5. May refer patients to private practitioners, the Local Authority paying an agreed fee.

The legal sanction for providing contraceptive treatment for married women in whose cases the avoidance of pregnancy is necessary to prevent aggravation of such existing organic diseases as tuberculosis, chronic nephritis, heart disease, etc., yet who are neither expectant nor nursing mothers nor suffering from some *gynæcological* condition, is to be found in Section 131 of the Public Health Act, 1875.[1]

> "Any local authority may provide for the use of the inhabitants of their district hospitals or temporary places for the reception of the sick, and for that purpose may—
>
> (1) Themselves build such hospital or part of a hospital or place of reception; or
> (2) Contract for the use of any such hospital or part of a hospital or place of reception; or
> (3) Enter into any agreement with any person having the management of any hospital, for the reception of the sick inhabitants of their district, on payment of such annual or other sum as may be agreed on."

At present, women suffering from organic diseases which constitute definite medical reasons for the avoidance of pregnancy, for whom no facilities for advice on birth control are provided by their Local Authorities, are dependent for information and instruction in methods of contraception upon:—

Hospitals.—The number of hospitals where advice is at present available is negligible.

Private Practitioners.—The uninsured woman may be prevented from consulting a doctor through reluctance or inability to pay the fee.

[1] This Act applies only to England and Wales. Scotland and Ireland have each a Public Health Act more or less resembling the 1875 Act.

Birth Control Centres maintained by private philanthropy.—The number and distribution of such clinics is quite inadequate to meet the need. (See list in Appendix.) At the clinics maintained by the Society for the Provision of Birth Control Clinics, a nominal consultation fee (one shilling) is charged, and appliances are sold at prices considerably below the current commercial rates. These clinics are staffed by qualified women doctors and trained nurses, and every patient is seen by the doctor in charge of the session.

A few Midwives and Unqualified Women who charge a small fee and who sell the necessary appliances.

Commercial firms and shops dealing in Contraceptive Devices.—The public has no protection against the sale of harmful or useless mechanical and chemical contraceptives: and in many cases the prices charged are exorbitant.

It is to be hoped that, in the near future, adequate provision for contraceptive advice and instruction for reasons of health will be included, together with the clinics for the prevention and treatment of rheumatism, cancer, tuberculosis, etc., among the health services of the country. Selective birth control should be an important branch of preventive medicine, for the reduction of maternal morbidity and mortality and for the promotion of child welfare.

Administration and Equipment of a Municipal Birth Control Clinic

The minimum equipment of a clinic for advice and instruction in methods of birth control is essentially the same as is required for an ante-natal clinic, with the addition of sets of occlusive pessaries for the fitting and instruction of patients, and a supply of occlusive pessaries, syringes, chemical contraceptives and sheaths for the patients' use. The " fitting pessaries " can be sterilised by boiling, and can be used repeatedly, over a period of months or years, according to the amount of wear and tear to which they are subjected and to their preservation when not in use. Rubber appliances, thoroughly dried and powdered with French chalk, may be stored in tins with close-fitting lids, in a cool place.

The exact arrangements of a clinic will depend largely upon the available premises and staff, and upon the number of patients to be dealt with. There must be facilities for :—

1. The accommodation of patients who are awaiting attention (waiting room or corridor).

2. The preparation of patients for the gynæcological examination (dressing room or cubicles and lavatory).

3. The medical examination, fitting and instruction in the use of a pessary (consulting room preferably with examination cubicles).

The general procedure may be as follows. Patients assemble in the waiting room, where the health visitor, nurse or lay worker may take the preliminary general history. If the desired particulars are already available on the patient's ante-natal or post-natal record card or on the gynæcological clinic record card, they may be copied on to a separate case paper. Some suitable modification of the case card reproduced may be used.

DATE.............................. No.

WALWORTH WOMEN'S WELFARE CENTRE

153A, EAST STREET, WALWORTH, S.E.17

Name ....

Address..

Heard of Centre from...

....

Date of Marriage........... Wife's Age...... Husband's Age.........

Husband's Occupation .... Wife's Occupation before marriage .... Wife's Occupation ....

Pregnancies..... Born alive..... Still born..... Miscarriages..... Alive now.....

Date.	Born Alive.	Still Born.	Miscarriages.	Sex.		Notes on Health or Death of Child, Miscarriage, Confinement, or Pregnancy.
1						
2						
3						
4						
5						
6						
7						
8						
9						
10						
11						
12						
13						
14						

Previous Methods.	Whether Adopted immediately on Marriage.	How Long Used.	Whether Effective.	Whether Satisfactory.	
				Husband.	Wife.
1 Abstinence . .					
2 Safe Period . .					
3 Coitus Interruptus .					
4 Sheath . . .					
5 Syringe . . .					
6 Rubber Pessary. .					
7 Sponge . . .					
8 Quinine Pessaries .					
9 Other Soluble Pessaries					
10 Post-Coital Micturition					
11 Prolonged Lactation .					
12 Any other Method .					

Front of Case Card.

Note.—The blank column, for recording previous attempts to procure abortions, and the space for particulars of birth control methods previously adopted, are included at the request of the Birth Control Investigation Committee.

Date General Condition
Bowels Micturition Periods Loss
Dysmenorrhœa Dyspareunia Last Menstrual Period
<u>On Examination</u> Vagina Perineum Cervix
Fundus Tubes Ovaries No. of Pessary
Ability to Learn

Date.	NOTES.

Back of Case Card.

Under the heading "No. of pessary," the full method of contraception advised is recorded.

Notes of subsequent visits, recording any changes in the local condition or in the method of birth control, are kept in the space below.

Following the name and address of the patient I would suggest " Referred for contraceptive advice by ...." and " Record of attendance at the Maternity and Child Welfare Centre or Gynæcological Clinic...................." When these preliminary particulars have been taken, the card should be transferred to the doctor's consulting room to be completed.

Before entering the doctor's room the patient should prepare for examination by removing clothing, emptying the bladder and lower bowel, and, finally, thoroughly washing the hands. For this purpose the use of a dressing room or cubicle, or a space screened off from the waiting room, and a lavatory with facilities for washing, are necessary.

The patient then proceeds to the doctor's consulting room, where the medical history is taken, and the medical indications for contraception are recorded. A gynæcological examination is made, and if an occlusive pessary be suitable, the patient is fitted with the correct size. The vaginal speculum, a selection of " fitting pessaries," and a bowl of lubricating fluid (soapy water containing a disinfectant) should be available on a conveniently placed shelf or table or trolley. For cases of abnormal dryness of the vagina, a tube of lubricating jelly, such as K-Y jelly, is useful. After the fitting the patient may be handed over to the nurse for instruction, or the doctor may herself instruct the patient in the insertion and removal of the pessary. It is an advantage to have two or more cubicles in the consulting room, each with examination couch and equipment, so that two or more patients may be receiving attention at the same time. Some patients learn to use the pessary correctly in five minutes; others need half an hour or more. At the Walworth Clinic there are five cubicles, so that five patients may be engaged simultaneously.

I recommend the procedure adopted at the clinics affiliated to the Society for the Provision of Birth Control Clinics. When the patient has succeeded in inserting and removing the pessary correctly three or four times, she is asked to practise adjusting the pessary at home at convenient times during the following week, and to return on a specified day, when she is asked to place the pessary in position so that it may be checked by the doctor. She is warned not to rely upon the pessary during the practice week, as not infrequently it is found, on her subsequent visit to the clinic, that she needs further instruction. She is therefore given the pessary only on her first visit; and on the second visit she is supplied with the remainder of her equipment, and instructed in the use of the syringe if syringing is advised. In some cases the doctor may decide that the routine second visit is unnecessary. If the patient is unwilling or unable to make the second visit special care is taken to ensure that she understands the proper use of the pessary, and extra instruction is given if necessary. In the few cases where the patient experiences great difficulty in learning the technique a third visit may be required in order that the doctor may feel assured of the patient's ability to use the appliance correctly.

The following printed instructions are supplied to clinic patients at the Walworth centre who are advised to use pessaries or sheaths :—

For Patients supplied with Occlusive Pessaries

IMPORTANT NOTES

1. Please return a week after your first visit, with the pessary in position, so that the doctor can tell you if you are placing it correctly.

2. The pessary, when new, is round, but tends to get out of shape. Gently press into a round shape before use.

3. Take care not to be constipated. If you are, the pessary is liable to fail.

4. Always smear the rim of the pessary on both sides with the jelly or ointment before use. Do not use vaseline or any other greasy ointment, as grease spoils rubber.

5. Never leave the pessary in for more than 12 hours.

6. Syringe before you take the pessary out with at least a pint of warm soapy water or vinegar and water (two tablespoonfuls to the quart). Clean the syringe.

Take out the pessary and syringe again with some fresh warm solution.

7. After use, wash the pessary and powder it with French chalk.

8. Do not use the pessary if the rim has snapped.

9. Patients are asked to report back to the Centre every six months.

Directions for use of Washable Sheaths

The Sheath must always be put on before there is any Contact whatever

1. Test each time before use. The presence of any tiny hole can be found by blowing into it.

2. Roll the sheath before use.

3. It is desirable before putting the sheath on to lubricate the male organ with the special jelly supplied. This makes it more comfortable and less likely to tear.

4. Leave about three-quarters of an inch of the sheath overlapping beyond the tip of the male organ.

5. When the sheath is on it is desirable that the outside be lubricated as well.

6. A few minutes before intercourse it is advisable for the woman to put a soluble pessary into her front passage.

7. After intercourse, take care the sheath does not slip off during withdrawal.

8. The sheath should be examined after intercourse. If there is a hole, however tiny, the woman should either douche at once or insert another soluble pessary.

9. After use wash the sheath with soapy water, dry, and powder it.

10. Keep flat in box.

11. Do not use after date on box, even if apparently in good condition, as rubber perishes within a few months of manufacture. This is not always apparent before use.

Directions for use of Sheath

(*To be used once only*)

1. Test before use. The presence of any tiny hole can be determined by blowing into the sheath.

2. It is desirable before putting it on to grease the male organ with the special jelly supplied.

3. Leave about three-quarters of an inch of the sheath overlapping beyond the tip of the male organ.

4. When the sheath is on it is desirable that the outside be greased as well.

5. A few minutes before intercourse it is advisable for the woman to insert a soluble pessary.

6. The sheath should be examined after intercourse. If it is torn or in any way defective the woman should douche at once.

7. Do not use after two months from date of purchase even if apparently in good condition, as rubber perishes within a few months of manufacture. This is not always apparent before use.

Instruction Cards supplied to Patients

Method A

(Rubber Cap, Ointment or Jelly, Syringe)

1. Smear the rubber cap on both sides with ointment or jelly before use.

2. Insert cap at convenient moment before getting into bed.

3. Allow cap to remain in for a few hours at least after intercourse before removing. Do not leave it in longer than twelve hours.

4. When you are ready to take the cap out, prepare about a quart of warm syringing solution, either vinegar and water (two tablespoonfuls to the quart) or soapy water. Syringe with half of this *before* you remove the cap, and use the remainder of the fluid *after* the cap is removed. Wash, dry, and powder the cap.

5. Take care not to be constipated. If back passage is not empty at time of inserting cap, it is not always possible to place it in the correct position.

Method B

(Rubber Cap, Ointment or Jelly, and Soluble Pessary)

1. Smear the cap on both sides with ointment or jelly before use.

2. Insert cap at convenient moment before getting into bed.

3. Insert soluble pessary five to ten minutes before intercourse, while lying down.

4. Leave the cap in for at least ten hours before removing. After use, wash, dry, and powder it.

5. Take care not to be constipated. If back passage is not empty at time of inserting cap it is not always possible to place it in the correct position.

Method C

(Rubber Cap, Ointment or Jelly, Soluble Pessary, and Syringe)

1. Smear the cap on both sides with ointment or jelly before use.

2. Insert cap at convenient time before going to bed.

3. Insert soluble pessary five to ten minutes before intercourse, while lying down.

4. Allow cap to remain in for a few hours at least after intercourse before removing. Do not leave it in longer than twelve hours.

5. When you are ready to take the cap out prepare about a quart of warm syringing solution, either vinegar and water (two tablespoonfuls to the quart) or soapy water. Syringe with half of this *before* you remove the cap, and use the remainder of the fluid *after* the cap is removed. Wash, dry, and powder the cap.

6. Take care not to be constipated. If back passage is not empty at time of inserting cap it is not always possible to place it in the correct position.

Method D

(Rubber Cap and Mil-San)

1. Moisten the cap with water or lubricate with a little Mil-San gently squeezed out of the tube.

2. Insert cap at convenient time before going to bed.

3. Insert Mil-San jelly (see directions in packet) just before intercourse, while lying down.

4. Allow cap to remain in for at least a few hours after intercourse before removing. Do not leave it in longer than twelve hours.

5. Take care not to be constipated. If back passage is not empty at time of inserting cap, it is not always possible to place it in the correct position.

Arrangements should be made for the renewal of appliances as required, and for subsequent visits to the clinic for a gynæcological examination at intervals of not less than six months. Changes in the patient's general health or local pelvic condition, or in her home circumstances, may indicate some change in the contraceptive method in use; and the harmlessness of the use of pessaries, syringes and chemical contraceptives should be confirmed at regular intervals.

For further details of the equipment of a birth control clinic the reader is referred to "On the Management of a Birth Control Centre," by Evelyn Fuller. Noel Douglas, price 1*s*. 6*d*.

Doctors and nurses who desire to be instructed in methods of birth control, and to observe the routine of a birth control clinic, should apply to the Secretary of the Society for the Provision of Birth Control Clinics, Walworth Women's Welfare Centre, East Street, Walworth, London, S.E.17. (See list of clinics in Appendix.)

APPENDIX

MINISTRY OF HEALTH MEMORANDUM 153/M.C.W. AND CIRCULAR 1208 [1]

For Official Use

MEMORANDUM 153/M.C.W.

Maternity and Child Welfare Authorities.

Birth Control

1. The Minister of Health is authorised to state that the Government have had under consideration the question of the use of institutions which are controlled by Local Authorities for the purpose of giving advice to women on contraceptive methods.

2. So far as Maternity and Child Welfare Centres (including Ante-Natal Centres) are concerned, these Centres can properly deal only with expectant mothers, nursing mothers, and young children, and it is the view of the Government that it is not the function of the Centres to give advice in regard to birth control and that their use for such a purpose would be likely to damage the proper work of the Centres. At the same time the Government consider that, in cases where there are ***medical grounds*** for giving advice on contraceptive methods to married women in attendance at the Centres, it may be given, but that such advice should be limited to ***cases where further pregnancy would be detrimental to health***, and should be given at a separate session and under conditions such as will not disturb the normal and primary work of the Centre. The Minister will accordingly be unable to sanction any proposal for the

[1] Reproduced by permission of the Controller of H.M. Stationery Office.

use of these Centres for giving birth control advice in other cases.

3. The Government are advised that Local Authorities have no general power to establish birth control clinics as such, but that under the Notification of Births (Extension) Act, 1915, which enables Local Authorities to exercise the powers of the Public Health Acts for the purpose of the care of expectant mothers and nursing mothers, it may properly be held that birth control clinics can be provided for these limited classes of women. Having regard to the acute division of public opinion on the subject of birth control, the Government have decided that no Departmental sanction which may be necessary to the establishment of such clinics for expectant and nursing mothers shall be given except on condition that contraceptive advice will be given only in *cases where further pregnancy would be detrimental to health.*

4. Under the Public Health Acts, Local Authorities have power to provide clinics at which medical advice and treatment would be available for women suffering from gynæcological conditions. But the enactments governing the provision of such clinics limit their availability to sick persons, and the Government have decided that any Departmental sanction which may be necessary to the establishment of such clinics shall be given only on the following conditions:—(1) that the clinics will be available only for women who are in need of medical advice and treatment for gynæcological conditions, and (2) that advice on contraceptive methods will be given only to married women who attend the clinics for such medical advice or treatment, *and in whose cases pregnancy would be detrimental to health.*

Ministry of Health.
March, 1931.

For Official Use

CIRCULAR 1208.[1]

Maternity and Child Welfare Authorities.

MINISTRY OF HEALTH,
Whitehall, London, S.W.1.
14th July, 1931.

Birth Control

SIR,

I am directed by the Minister of Health to refer to Memorandum 153/M.C.W., which was issued in March last on the above subject. The Minister finds that certain misconceptions have arisen in regard to the views expressed in that Memorandum, and he desires to bring the following points to the notice of Local Authorities.

1. It is necessary to emphasise the statement in the Memorandum that the Government are advised that Local Authorities have no general power to establish birth control clinics as such. The Memorandum was issued solely for the purpose of explaining the views of the Government on the use of institutions controlled by Local Authorities for the purpose of giving advice to women on contraceptive methods, and it should be understood that the question of providing facilities for giving such advice within the limits laid down in the Memorandum is a matter entirely within the discretion of the Local Authority.

2. Under the Maternity and Child Welfare Act, 1918, the powers of Local Authorities are limited, so far as women are concerned, to making arrangements for attending to the health of expectant mothers and nursing mothers. If an Authority decides to provide facilities for giving birth control advice at a Maternity and Child Welfare Centre in accordance with paragraph 2 of the Memorandum, the use of these facilities must be strictly incidental to the purpose for which the Centre is established, and they can be made available

[1] Reproduced by permission of the Controller of H.M. Stationery Office.

only for married women who are either expectant or nursing mothers already in attendance at the Centre and in whose cases further pregnancy would be detrimental to health.

3. If action is taken under the Public Health Acts to establish a clinic at which medical advice and treatment would be available for women suffering from gynæcological conditions, the use of any facilities provided at the clinic for giving advice on contraceptive methods must be strictly incidental to the purpose for which the clinic is established, viz., the treatment of sick persons. Only women who need medical advice and treatment for gynæcological conditions can properly be admitted to the clinic, and contraceptive advice can properly be given only to married women in attendance at the clinic in whose cases pregnancy would be detrimental to health. It is obviously desirable for a Local Authority to obtain the services of a medical officer specially experienced in the clinical advice and treatment needed at a gynæcological centre of this sort.

4. The Minister does not consider it desirable that a gynæcological clinic should be established at a Maternity and Child Welfare Centre, and if an Authority is satisfied that there is need for such a clinic it should be provided in separate premises or at a hospital. Expectant mothers and nursing mothers in attendance at Maternity and Child Welfare Centres who are found to need medical advice and treatment for gynæcological conditions could then be referred to the clinic.

5. The Minister considers it important that no existing officer of a Local Authority should be prejudiced in any way by a decision of the Authority to provide facilities for birth control advice within the limits laid down in the Memorandum. He is of opinion that this work should not be regarded as falling within the scope of the normal duties of the medical officers of a Local Authority who should be free to undertake it or decline it.

I am, Sir,

Your obedient Servant,

A. K. MACLACHLEN,

Assistant Secretary.

The Clerk to the Local Authority.

CIRCULAR 1408.[1]

Maternity and Child Welfare Authorities.

MINISTRY OF HEALTH,
Whitehall, London, S.W.1.
31*st May*, 1934.

Birth Control

SIR,

1. I am directed by the Minister of Health to refer to Memorandum 153/M.C.W. dated March, 1931, and Circular 1208 of the 14th July, 1931, and more particularly to paragraph 4 of the Memorandum and paragraph 3 of the Circular which deal with the provision under the Public Health Acts of clinics for women suffering from gynæcological conditions. It was stated in paragraph 4 of the Memorandum that the Government had decided that any Departmental sanction which might be necessary to the establishment of such clinics should be given only on condition :—

(1) that the clinics will be available only for women who are in need of medical advice and treatment for gynæcological conditions and (2) that advice on contraceptive methods will be given only to married women who attend the clinics for such medical advice or treatment, and in whose cases pregnancy would be detrimental to health.

2. The Authority will be aware that the Departmental Committee on Maternal Mortality and Morbidity, in their Final Report published in 1932, called special attention to the importance of the avoidance of pregnancy by women suffering from organic disease such as tuberculosis, heart disease, diabetes, chronic nephritis, etc., in which childbearing is likely seriously to endanger life. The Committee considered that advice and instruction in contraceptive methods should be readily available for such women.

3. It was pointed out in the Memorandum and Circular of 1931 that the powers which the Public Health Acts confer upon Local Authorities for the provision of clinics limit their availability to sick persons, but the Minister is advised that there is

[1] Reproduced by permission of H.M. Stationery Office.

nothing to prevent the Local Authority from rendering such a clinic available for women suffering from forms of sickness other than gynæcological conditions. After careful consideration of the recommendation made by the Departmental Committee, the Minister is of opinion that where a Local Authority has provided a clinic at which medical advice and treatment are available for married women suffering from gynæcological conditions, and at which contraceptive advice is afforded to married women so suffering in whose cases pregnancy would be detrimental to health, it would be proper also for married women who are suffering from other forms of sickness, physical or mental, such as those mentioned in the Report of the Departmental Committee, which are detrimental to them as mothers, to be afforded contraceptive advice at the clinic if it is found medically that pregnancy would be detrimental to health. What is, or is not, medically detrimental to health must be decided by the professional judgment of the registered medical practitioner in charge of the clinic.

I am, Sir,

Your obedient Servant,

A. K. MACLACHLEN,

Assistant Secretary.

The Clerk to the Local Authority.

The Department of Health for Scotland have issued no statement defining the powers of the Scottish Public Health Authorities to provide information and instruction on birth control. The Notification of Births (Extension) Act, 1915, applies also to Scotland; so that presumably facilities for birth control advice and instruction may be provided for expectant and nursing mothers who are attending institutions under the control of the Local Authorities, and in whose cases there are medical grounds for the prevention or postponement of further pregnancies.

ACTION TAKEN BY LOCAL AUTHORITIES UNDER MINISTRY OF HEALTH MEMORANDUM 153/M.C.W., CIRCULAR 1208/M.C.W. AND CIRCULAR 1408/M.C.W.

These particulars are kindly supplied by the Secretary of the National Birth Control Association.

LOCAL AUTHORITIES who have taken action to provide facilities for giving advice on Birth Control under the Ministry of Health Memorandum 153/M.C.W., Circular 1208/M.C.W., and Circular 1408/M.C.W.

1. The following Local Authorities have established clinics where birth control advice is given, usually in connection with Maternity and Child Welfare Centres:—

Aberavon and Port Talbot M. B.
Aberdare U. D. C.
Barnes M. B.
Barrow-in-Furness C. B.
Bath City C.
Batley M. B.
Bethnal Green Met. B.
Birmingham City C.
Blackpool C. B.
Bournemouth C. B.
Brighton C. B.
Burton-on-Trent C. B.
Caerphilly U. D. C.
Chelmsford M. B.
Colwyn Bay M. B.
Crewe M. B.
Dartford M. B.
Dewsbury C. B.
Dudley C. B.
Durham C. C. (six centres).
Ealing M. B.
Essex C. C. (seven centres).
Gellygaer U. D. C.
Gillingham M. B.
Gloucestershire C. C.
Gloucester City C.
Grimsby C. B.
Halifax C. B.
Harrow U. D. C.
Kendal M. B.
Leicester City C.
Lincoln C. B.
Llantrisant R. D. C.
Mexborough U. D. C.
Mountain Ash U. D. C. (three centres).
Norwich City C.
Ogmore and Garw U. D. C.
Portsmouth M. B.
Reigate M. B.
Rhondda U. D. C.
Rotherham C. B.
Southgate M. B.
Stoke Newington M. B.
Stoke-on-Trent C. B.
Wembley U. D. C.
West Hartlepool C. B.
West Riding (Yorks.) C. C. (three centres).
York City C.

2. The following have set up Gynæcological Clinics at which birth control advice is given :—

Barry U. D. C.
Bristol City C.
Croydon M. B.
Doncaster C. B.
Fulham Met. B.
Hull City C.
Leeds City C.
Manchester City C. (two centres).
Oxford City C.
Penarth U. D. C.
Pontypridd U. D. C.
St. Helens C. B.
Sheffield City C.
Shoreditch Met. B.
Southampton C. B. (two centres).
Sunderland C. B.
Tilbury U. D. C.
Walthamstow M. B.
West Bromwich C. B.
West Riding (Yorks.) C. C. (one centre).

3. The following refer cases to voluntary or municipal clinics or private doctors :

(*a*) paying a fee for each patient :—

Acton M. B.
Aldershot M. B.
Ashington U. D. C.
Banbury M. B.
Bedford M. B.
Bedlington U. D. C.
Buckinghamshire C. C.
Cambridge M. B.
Cambridgeshire C. C.
Cheltenham M. B.
Dagenham U. D. C.
Denbighshire C. C.
Devonshire C. C.
Durham C. C.
Edmonton U. D. C.
Exeter City C.
Gloucestershire C. C.
Glyncorrwg U. D. C.
Greenwich Met. B.
Hampshire C. C.
Hebburn U. D. C.
Hove M. B.
Leicestershire C. C.
Lytham St. Annes M. B.
Middlesex C. C.
Newburn U. D. C.
Norfolk C. C.
Northamptonshire C. C.
Northumberland C. C.
Nottingham City C.
Nuneaton M. B.
Paddington Met. B.
Plymouth City C.
Rochdale C. B.
Romford U. D. C.
Salford City C.
Somerset C. C.
Stretford M. B.
Sussex (East) C. C.
Sussex (West) C. C.
Swinton (Lancs.) M. B.
Torquay M. B.
Wandsworth Met. B.
West Ham C. B.

(*b*) making a block grant :—

Aberdeen M. B.
Kensington Royal Boro'
Leeds City C.
Liverpool City C.
Newcastle City C.
Northampton C. B.
Renfrew Royal Burgh.
Sheffield City C.
Southall U. D. C.
Tynemouth C. B.
Willesden M. B.
Worcestershire C. C.

4. The following have authorised their Medical Officers to give advice, but have started no special clinics :—

Blyth M. B.
Chester M. B.
Christchurch M. B.
Coventry C. B.
Darlington M. B.
Dover M. B.
Enfield U. D. C.
Flintshire C. C.
Hartlepool M. B.
Heston and Isleworth M. B.
Hornsey M. B.
Hyde M. B.
Ilkley U. D. C.
Keighley M. B.
Loughborough M. B.
Mansfield M. B.
Mansfield Woodhouse U. D. C.
Market Harborough U. D. C.
Marylebone Met. B.
Merton and Morden U. D. C.
Middlesbrough C. B.
Oldham C. B.
Paignton U. D. C.
Ramsgate M. B.
Retford (East) M. B.
Royton U. D. C.
Sevenoaks U. D. C.
South Shields C. B.
Teddington U. D. C.
Wakefield City C.
Walsall C. B.
Wednesbury M. B.
Westminster Met. B.
Wombwell U. D. C.
Worthing M. B.

5. The following have decided to give advice, and are either now considering schemes or have not yet taken steps to put the decision into effect :—

Blackburn C. B.
Canterbury C. B.
Carlisle C. B.
Colne M. B.
Cumberland C. C.
Hammersmith Met. B.
Lancashire C. C.
Llanelly M. B.
Pontardawe R. D. C.
Poplar Met. B.
Southport C. B.
Twickenham M. B.
Workington M. B.
Warwickshire C. C.

6. The following have either lent or hired the premises of a Maternity and Child Welfare Centre to a local branch of the National Birth Control Association, or similar body, for use as a voluntary birth control clinic :—

Aldershot M. B.
Ashington U. D. C.
Barnstaple M. B.
Cambridge M. B.
Dagenham U. D. C.
Derby C. B.
Greenock (Parl. B.).
Guildford M. B.
Hampshire C. C.
Northampton C. B.
Portsmouth City C.
Plymouth C. B.
Sheffield M. B.
Willesden M. B.
Winchester M. B.

C. B. = County Borough. M. B. = Municipal Borough. C. C. = County Council. U. D. C. = Urban District Council.

There are 1,846 Local (Public Health) Authorities in England and Wales, of whom over 400 maintain maternity and infant welfare centres.

BIRTH CONTROL CLINICS

Clinics affiliated to the Society for the Provision of Birth Control Clinics[1]

All fittings are done by a qualified woman doctor, who is present throughout each session to examine and advise patients.

London and District

Affiliated Centres.	Hours of Attendance.
CROYDON BIRTH CONTROL CLINIC, 33, St. James' Road, Croydon, Surrey.	Second and Fourth Wednesday in the month, 2.30–4.0 p.m.
DAGENHAM AND DISTRICT BIRTH CONTROL CLINIC, The Clinic, Becontree Avenue, Dagenham, Essex.	Second and Fourth Thursday in the month, 7.0–9.0 p.m.

[1] Before referring patients to these clinics it is advisable to write to the Secretary of the Society, Walworth Women's Welfare Centre, for latest particulars of addresses and times of sessions, as these may be changed from time to time.

London and District—*Continued.*

Affiliated Centres.	Hours of Attendance.
EAST LONDON WOMEN'S WELFARE CENTRE, 6, BURDETT ROAD, STEPNEY, E.3.	Monday and Wednesday, 2.30–4.0 p.m.
GOSWELL WOMEN'S WELFARE CENTRE, 39, SPENCER STREET, GOSWELL ROAD, E.C.1.	Monday, 6.30–8.30 p.m. Thursday, 2.30–4.0 p.m. Gynæcological Clinic, Friday, 7.30–8.30 p.m.
GREENWICH WOMEN'S WELFARE ASSOCIATION, 118, WOOLWICH ROAD, GREENWICH, S.E.10.	Thursday, 2.0–4.0 p.m.
NORTH KENSINGTON WOMEN'S WELFARE CENTRE, 12, TELFORD ROAD, LADBROKE GROVE, W.10.	Monday and Friday, 2.30–4.0 p.m. Tuesday and Wednesday, 6.30–8.0 p.m. Gynæcological Clinic, Tuesday, 6.30–8.0 p.m. Thursday, 2.0–3.30 p.m. Friday, 2.30–4.0 p.m.
SOUTH-WEST LONDON WOMEN'S WELFARE CENTRE, BATTERSEA CHAPEL SCHOOL HALL, YORK ROAD, BATTERSEA, S.W.	Tuesday, 2.0–4.0 p.m.
WALWORTH WOMEN'S WELFARE CENTRE, 153A, EAST STREET, S.E.17.	Tuesday and Friday, 2.30–4.0 p.m. Thursday, 6.30–8.0 p.m.
WILLESDEN WOMEN'S WELFARE CENTRE, MUNICIPAL HEALTH CENTRE (1), 9, WILLESDEN LANE, KILBURN, N.W.6.	Wednesday, 6.30–8.0 p.m.

Provinces

ALDERSHOT AND DISTRICT WOMEN'S WELFARE CENTRE, MANOR HOUSE CLINIC, MANOR PARK, ALDERSHOT, HANTS.	First two Tuesdays in the month, 3.0–5.0 p.m.
ASHINGTON AND DISTRICT BIRTH CONTROL CLINIC, CHILD WELFARE CENTRE, SOUTH VIEW, ASHINGTON, NORTHUMBERLAND.	Last Friday in the month, 2.30–4.0 p.m.

Provinces—*Continued.*

Affiliated Centres.	Hours of Attendance.
BASINGSTOKE AND DISTRICT MOTHERS' CLINIC, CASTONS ROAD, BASINGSTOKE, HANTS.	Alternate Fridays, 2.30–4.0 p.m. Apply to Secretary.
BIRKENHEAD MOTHERS' WELFARE CLINIC, 11A, OXTON ROAD, BIRKENHEAD, CHESHIRE.	Tuesday, 2.0–3.0 p.m. Thursday, 6.0–7.0 p.m.
BIRMINGHAM WOMEN'S WELFARE CENTRE, 22, MASSHOUSE LANE, NEAR MOOR STREET AND ALBERT STREET, BIRMINGHAM, WARWICKSHIRE.	Monday and Thursday, 2.30–4.0 p.m. Tuesday, 7.30–9.0 p.m.
BRISTOL MOTHERS' WELFARE CENTRE, SALFORD HALL, ST. JAMES' BARTON, BRISTOL, GLOS.	Friday, 10.0–12 noon.
CAMBRIDGE WOMEN'S WELFARE ASSOCIATION, 22, PARSONAGE STREET, CAMBRIDGE (OFF NEWMARKET ROAD, BEHIND THE STAR BREWERY), CAMBS.	Wednesday, 3.0–5.0 p.m.
DERBY MOTHERS' CLINIC, MATERNITY AND CHILD WELFARE ROOMS, NIGHTINGALE ROAD (Amber Street Entrance), DERBY, DERBYSHIRE.	Second and Fourth Thursday in the month, 7.30–8.30 p.m.
EAST KENT MARRIED WOMEN'S ADVISORY CLINIC, 24, GILFORD ROAD, DEAL, KENT. (Entrance, Grove Road.)	Second and Fourth Wednesday in the month, 3.0–4.30 p.m.
EXETER AND DISTRICT WOMEN'S WELFARE ASSOCIATION, THE DISPENSARY, QUEEN STREET, EXETER, DEVON.	Friday, 2.15–5.0 p.m.
BRANCH AT: DARTINGTON, TOTNES, DEVON.	Apply to Secretary at Exeter.
GRIMSBY WOMEN'S WELFARE CLINIC, WATKIN STREET HALL, GRIMSBY, LINCS.	Monday, 2.30–4.0 p.m.
GUILDFORD WOMEN'S WELFARE CENTRE, 6, STOKE ROAD, GUILDFORD, SURREY.	First two Wednesdays in the month, 5.0 p.m.

Provinces—*Continued.*

Affiliated Centres.	Hours of Attendance.
HALIFAX WOMEN'S WELFARE CLINIC, 19, SAVILE ROAD, HALIFAX, YORKS.	Second and Fourth Wednesday in the month, 7.0–8.30 p.m.
HEREFORD WOMEN'S WELFARE CENTRE, 1, CARLTON FLATS, EIGN STREET, HEREFORD.	Wednesday, 2.0–3.30 p.m.
LIVERPOOL MOTHERS' WELFARE CLINIC, 23, CLARENCE STREET, OFF MOUNT PLEASANT, LIVERPOOL, 3, LANCS.	Wednesday, 2.0–3.0 p.m. Friday, 6.30–7.30 p.m.
BRANCH AT: COMMUNITY HALL, TOWNSEND AVENUE, NORRIS GREEN, LIVERPOOL, 11, LANCS.	Monday, 2.0–3.0 p.m.
MANCHESTER, SALFORD, AND DISTRICT MOTHERS' CLINIC FOR BIRTH CONTROL, 123, GREENGATE, SALFORD, LANCS. (Entrance, Garden Lane.)	Thursday, 3.0 p.m. and 7.30 p.m.
MEDWAY TOWNS MOTHERS' ADVICE CENTRE, HENDERSON HOUSE, NEW ROAD, ROCHESTER, KENT.	Last two Tuesdays in the month, 2.30–4.0 p.m.
NEWCASTLE WOMEN'S WELFARE CENTRE, 24, SHIELDFIELD GREEN, NEWCASTLE-ON-TYNE, NORTHUMBERLAND.	Tuesday and Thursday, 2.30–4.0 p.m.
NORTHAMPTON WOMEN'S WELFARE ASSOCIATION, APPLY SECRETARY, 5, CASTILIAN TERRACE, NORTHAMPTON.	Third Thursday in the month, 6.30–8.30 p.m. Fourth Thursday in the month, 6.30–7.30 p.m.
NORTH DEVON WOMEN'S WELFARE AND ADVICE CENTRE, 113, BOUTPORT STREET, BARNSTAPLE, DEVON.	Apply to Hon. Secretary for times of attendance.
NORTH STAFFORDSHIRE MOTHERS' ADVICE CLINIC, 12, WELLESLEY STREET, HOWARD PLACE, SHELTON, STOKE-ON-TRENT, STAFFS.	First and Third Monday in the month, 2.30–4.0 p.m. (Opened November, 1936.)
NOTTINGHAM WOMEN'S WELFARE ASSOCIATION, 15, MARKET STREET, NOTTINGHAM, NOTTS.	Thursday, 2.30–4.30 p.m.

Provinces—*Continued.*

Affiliated Centres.	Hours of Attendance.
OXFORD FAMILY WELFARE ASSOCIATION, 4, KING STREET, JERICHO, OXFORD, OXON.	Wednesday, 2.30–4.0 p.m. (Women) Men: By appointment.
PLYMOUTH MOTHERS' ADVICE CENTRE, BEAUMONT HUT, BEAUMONT PARK, PLYMOUTH, DEVON.	Tuesday, 6.45–9.0 p.m.
PORTSMOUTH WOMEN'S WELFARE CENTRE, TRAFALGAR PLACE (CLIVE ROAD), FRATTON ROAD, PORTSMOUTH.	Tuesday, 6.0–8.0 p.m.
SALISBURY MARRIED WOMEN'S ADVISORY CLINIC, 49, HIGH STREET, SALISBURY, WILTS.	First and Third Thursday in the month, 2.0–4.0 p.m.
SHEFFIELD WOMEN'S WELFARE CLINIC, ATTERCLIFFE VESTRY HALL, ATTERCLIFFE COMMON, SHEFFIELD, 9, YORKS.	Every Tuesday, 6.0–8.0 p.m. and First Tuesday in the month, 2.30–4.0 p.m.
SHILDON AND DISTRICT MOTHERS' CLINIC, 2, MARKET PLACE, SHILDON, CO. DURHAM.	Thursday, 2.30–4.0 p.m. (Opened October, 1936.)
SLOUGH AND DISTRICT MARRIED WOMEN'S ADVISORY CLINIC, 272, FARNHAM ROAD, SLOUGH, BUCKS.	Wednesday, 2.30–4.0 p.m.
STAFFORDSHIRE AND DISTRICT WOMEN'S WELFARE CENTRE, 62, HEATH STREET, HEATH TOWN, WOLVERHAMPTON, STAFFS.	First Wednesday in the month, 2.0–4.0 p.m.
SUNDERLAND WOMEN'S ADVISORY CLINIC, 46, JOHN STREET, SUNDERLAND, CO. DURHAM.	Second and Third Wednesday in the month, 2.0–4.30 p.m.
TYNEMOUTH AND DISTRICT WOMEN'S ADVISORY CENTRE, 1, CLEVELAND ROAD (OFF PRESTON ROAD), NORTH SHIELDS, NORTHUMBERLAND.	Every Tuesday, 2.0–4.0 p.m. and First and Second Tuesday in the month, 7.0–8.0 p.m.

Provinces—*Continued.*

Affiliated Centres.	Hours of Attendance.
WELWYN GARDEN CITY MARRIED WOMEN'S CLINIC, LAWRENCE HALL, APPLECROFT ROAD, WELWYN GARDEN CITY, HERTS.	Second and Fourth Friday in the month, 7.30–9.0 p.m.
WINCHESTER AND DISTRICT MARRIED WOMEN'S ADVISORY CLINIC, 4, THE SQUARE, WINCHESTER, HANTS.	Second and Fourth Thursday in the month, 2.0–3.30 p.m.

Scotland

DUNDEE MOTHERS' WELFARE ADVISORY CLINIC, HILLSIDE WORKS HALL, 114, HILLTOWN, DUNDEE, ANGUS.	Tuesday, 3.0–4.30 p.m. (Opened October, 1936.)
EDINBURGH MOTHERS' WELFARE CLINIC, 90, EAST CROSSCAUSEWAY, EDINBURGH, 8, MIDLOTHIAN.	Tuesday, 6.30–8.0 p.m. Friday, 2.0–3.0 p.m.
BRANCH : CRAIGMILLAR COLLEGE, UNIVERSITY SETTLEMENT, NIDDRIE.	Friday, 6.0–7.0 p.m.
GLASGOW WOMEN'S WELFARE AND ADVISORY CLINIC, 123, MONTROSE STREET, GLASGOW, C.4, LANARKSHIRE.	Tuesday, 7.0–8.0 p.m. Thursday, 3.0–4.0 p.m.
GREENOCK BIRTH CONTROL CLINIC, MATERNITY & CHILD WELFARE CENTRE, TERRACE ROAD, GREENOCK, RENFREWSHIRE.	Apply to Secretary.
PAISLEY MOTHERS' CLINIC, BANK STREET, CO-OPERATIVE HALL, PAISLEY, RENFREWSHIRE.	Tuesday, 7.0–8.0 p.m.

Wales

MERTHYR COUNTY BOROUGH VOLUNTARY BIRTH CONTROL CLINIC, GLEBELAND STREET CLINIC, MERTHYR TYDVIL, GLAMORGANSHIRE.	Alternate Fridays, 11 a.m. Apply Secretary.

Society for Constructive Birth Control and Racial Progress

Patients are seen by a qualified nurse, who may refer them to the clinic doctor if she considers it advisable to do so.

FREE CLINICS FOR CONSTRUCTIVE BIRTH CONTROL
(Founded by Dr. M. C. Stopes and Captain H. V. Roe.)

Affiliated Centres.	Hours of Attendance.
1. MOTHERS' CLINIC, 108, WHITFIELD STREET, TOTTENHAM COURT ROAD, LONDON, W.1.	Monday to Friday, 10.0 a.m.–6.0 p.m.
2. LEEDS, 68, BELLEVUE ROAD.	Monday to Friday, 10.0 a.m.–6.0 p.m.
3. ABERDEEN, 4, GERRARD STREET, GALLOWGATE, ABERDEEN, SCOTLAND.	Monday to Friday, 10.0 a.m.–6.0 p.m.
4. BELFAST C.B.C. CLINIC, 103, THE MOUNT, BELFAST.	Monday to Friday, 10.0 a.m. to 6.0 p.m.

CONTRACEPTIVES

Only those chemical contraceptives of which the constituents have been divulged by the manufacturers are listed.

SUPPOSITORIES

"Chinobut" (chinosol). Lamberts Prorace Ltd.
"Lam-Butt" (quinine). Lamberts Prorace Ltd.
Lactic acid pessaries. Martindale.
[1] "G.P." solubles. Gilmont Products Ltd.
"Prentif" cocoa-butter. Prentif Ltd.
"Prentif" gelatine (large). Prentif Ltd.
[1] "Prensols" gelatine (small). Prentif Ltd.
"Proseldis" suppositories. Proseldis Chemical Co.
"Racial" suppositories. Society of Constructive Birth Control and Racial Products.
Rendell's suppositories. W. J. Rendell.
"Vimule" suppositories. A. Lambert & Sons.

JELLIES AND OINTMENTS

Contraceptalene. Lamberts Prorace Ltd.
Durol. London Rubber Co.
"Eugam" contraceptive jelly. Harman Freese.

[1] Prepared for use with occlusive pessaries only.

Freelac jelly. Proseldis Chemical Co.
G.P. jelly. Gilmont Products Ltd.
G.P. ointment. Gilmont Products Ltd.
K.Y. lubricating jelly. Johnson & Johnson.
" Koromex " vaginal jelly. Prentif Ltd.
Mil-San jelly. Menosine Ltd.
Ortho-Gynol jelly. Johnson & Johnson.
PermFoam. Gilmont Products Ltd.
" Prentif " lubricating jelly. Prentif Ltd.
" Prentif " spermicidal compound. Prentif Ltd.
" Proseldis " jelly. Proseldis Chemical Co.
Spetonex jelly. Coates & Cooper.
Van de Velde's contraceptive jelly. Harman Freese.

FOAM TABLETS
Antipart. Francis O. Rudloph-Riddell.
Bircon. London Rubber Co.
Bymeston. Lamberts Prorace Ltd.
" Hygena " contraceptive tablets. A. Lambert & Sons.
Lomolo. H. R. Napp Ltd.
" Proseldis " effervescing tablets. Proseldis Chemical Co.
Semori. Medical Laboratories Ltd.
Speton. Coates & Cooper Ltd.

OCCLUSIVE PESSARIES
Allen & Hanburys.
Harman Freese.
A. Lambert & Sons.
Lamberts Prorace Ltd.
London Rubber Co.
Prentif Ltd.
Proseldis Chemical Co.
Surgical Manufacturing Co. Ltd.

STEM PESSARIES
Allen & Hanburys Ltd.
Surgical Manufacturing Co. Ltd.

INTRA-UTERINE (GRÄFENBERG) RING
Allen & Hanburys Ltd.
Surgical Manufacturing Co. Ltd.

LIST OF MANUFACTURERS OR AGENTS

ALLEN & HANBURYS LTD., 48, Wigmore Street, London, W.1.
Dutch pessaries.
Cervical caps.
" Wishbone " gold spring stem pessaries.
Gräfenberg intra-uterine ring, introducer and removing hook.

COATES & COOPER LTD., 94, Clerkenwell Road, London, E.C.1.
Speton foam tablets.
Spetonex jelly.

HARMAN FREESE, 32, Great Dover Street, London, S.E.1.
Van de Velde's contraceptives:
" Gamophile " occlusive pessaries (Dutch, Retroflexion, Hodge-Smith model, and cervical cap).
" Eugam " contraceptive jelly.
" Eugam " lubricating jelly.

GILMONT PRODUCTS LTD., Tileyard Road, York Road, London, N.7.
G.P.D. (douche).
G.P. jelly.
G.P. ointment.
G.P. solubles.
PermFoam foaming jelly.

JOHNSON & JOHNSON, Slough, Bucks.
K.Y. lubricating jelly.
Ortho-Gynol jelly.

LAMBERT & SONS, 16, Dalston Lane, London, E.8.
" Vimule " suppositories (quinine).
" Vimule " suppositories (chinosol).
" Hygena " contraceptive tablets.
Occlusive pessaries (diaphragm, vault and cervical caps).

LAMBERTS PRORACE LTD., 60, Queen's Road, Dalston, London, E.8.
" Chinobut " suppositories (chinosol).
" Lam-Butt " suppositories (quinine).
Contraceptalene jelly.
Bymeston foam tablets.
Occlusive pessaries (Dutch, Dumas and Pro-race).
Dutch with watch-spring rim.
Dutch with " Duplex " rim (spiral enclosing watch-spring).
Dumas—ordinary heavy white rubber.
Dumas—*soft* brown rubber.

LONDON RUBBER CO., Elarco House, 221, Old Street, London, E.C.1.
Bircon foam tablets.
Condoms and sheaths.
Durol lubricating jelly.
Occlusive pessaries (Dutch and Elarco check).

W. MARTINDALE, 12, New Cavendish Street, London, W.1.
Lactic acid suppositories.
Quinine suppositories.

MEDICAL LABORATORIES LTD., 40, Pall Mall, London, S.W.1.
Lactic acid pessaries.
Semori foam tablets.

MENOSINE LTD., 24, Maple Street, London, W.1.
Mil-San jelly.

H. R. NAPP LTD., 3, Clement's Inn, Kingsway, London, W.C.2.
Lomolo foam tablets.

PARKE, DAVIS & Co., Beak Street, Regent Street, London, W.C.1.
Quinine urea hydrochloride tablets.

PRENTIF LTD., Long's Court, St. Martin's Street, London, W.C.2.
"Prentif" condoms and washable sheaths (dated goods).
Cervical caps and Dumas-type caps.
"Prentif" gelatine suppositories and "Prensols."
Agents for Holland-Rantos Company Inc., New York.
"Koromex" diaphragms.
"Koromex" vaginal jelly.

PROSELDIS CHEMICAL Co., 32, Great Dover Street, London, S.E.1.
"Proseldis" effervescing tablets.
"Proseldis" suppositories.
"Proseldis" birth control jelly.
"Freelac" jelly.
"Proseldis" douching pellets.
Dutch pessaries.

W. J. RENDELL, Hardwick House, Rosebery Avenue, London, E.C.
Rendell's pessaries.

RUDLOPH-RIDDELL, FRANCIS O., Sentinel House, Southampton Row, London, W.C.1.
Antipart foam tablets.

SOCIETY OF CONSTRUCTIVE BIRTH CONTROL AND RACIAL PRODUCTS, 108, Whitfield Street, London, W.1.
"Racial" suppositories, "Racial" occlusive pessaries, "Racial" sponges.

SURGICAL MANUFACTURING Co. LTD., 83–85, Mortimer Street, London, W.1.
Cervical caps.
Gräfenberg intra-uterine ring.
Stem pessaries.

BIBLIOGRAPHY

CHARLES, E. " The Practice of Birth Control," 1932. Williams & Norgate.

COOPER, J. F. " Technique of Contraception," 1928. Day-Nichols, New York.

DAVIS, K. BEMENT. " Factors in the Sex Life of Twenty-two Hundred Women," 1929. Harper & Brothers, New York and London.

DEPARTMENTAL COMMITTEE ON MORTALITY AND MORBIDITY, MINISTRY OF HEALTH. Interim and Final Reports, 1930, 1932. His Majesty's Stationery Office.

DICKINSON, R. L., and LURA BEAM. " A Thousand Marriages," 1931. Williams & Wilkins Co., Baltimore, U.S.A.

DICKINSON, R. L., and L. S. BRYANT. " Control of Conception," 1932. Baillière, Tindall & Cox, London.

INTERNATIONAL MEDICAL GROUP FOR THE INVESTIGATION OF CONTRACEPTION. Third and Fourth Reports, 1930, 1931. C. P. Blacker. Birth Control Investigation Committee, London.

EDEN, T. W., and E. L. HOLLAND. " Manual of Midwifery," 1931. J. & A. Churchill, London.

FULLER, EVELYN. " On the Management of a Birth Control Centre." Noel Douglas, London.

HARTMAN, CARL G. " Time of Ovulation in Women," 1936. Baillière, Tindall & Cox, London.

HIMES, NORMAN E. " Medical History of Contraception," 1936. G. Allen & Unwin Ltd.

KONIKOW, A. F. " Physicians' Manual of Birth Control," 1931. Baillière, Tindall & Cox, London.

MALLESON, JOAN. " The Principles of Contraception," 1935. Gollancz.

REPORTS OF THE INTERNATIONAL MEDICAL GROUP FOR THE INVESTIGATION OF CONTRACEPTION (five issues). Birth Control Investigation Committee, 26, Eccleston Street, S.W.1.

ROBSON, J. M. " Recent Advances in Sex and Reproductive Physiology," 1934. J. & A. Churchill.

SANGER, M., and H. M. STONE. " The Practice of Contraception," 1931. Baillière, Tindall & Cox, London.

STOPES, M. C. " Contraception," Third Edition, 1931. G. P. Putnam's Sons, London.

VAN DE VELDE, TH. H. " Fertility and Sterility in Marriage," 1931. Heinemann (Medical Books) Ltd., London.

VAN DE VELDE, TH. H. " Ideal Marriage," 1932. Heinemann (Medical Books) Ltd., London.

VOGE, I. B. " The Chemistry and Physics of Contraceptives," 1933. Jonathan Cape, London.

WALKER, K. " Male Disorders of Sex," 1930. Jonathan Cape, London.

Birth Control Organisations

1. THE NATIONAL BIRTH CONTROL ASSOCIATION, 26, Eccleston Street, S.W.1.
   President : Lord Horder, K.C.V.O., M.D., F.R.C.P.
   Chairman of Executive Committee : Lady Denman, D.B.E.

2. THE BIRTH CONTROL INVESTIGATION COMMITTEE, 26, Eccleston Street, S.W.1.
   Chairman of Executive Committee : Sir Humphrey Rolleston, Bart., G.C.V.O., K.C.B., M.D., M.R.C.P.
   Hon. Secretary : Dr. C. P. Blacker, M.D., M.R.C.P.

3. THE SOCIETY FOR THE PROVISION OF BIRTH CONTROL CLINICS, 153A, East Street, Walworth, S.E.17.
   Chairman of Executive Committee : Lord Gerald Wellesley.
   Secretary : Mrs. Evelyn Fuller.

4. THE SOCIETY FOR CONSTRUCTIVE BIRTH CONTROL, 108, Whitfield Street, W.1.
   President : Dr. Marie Stopes, D.Sc., D.Ph.

5. THE BIRTH CONTROL INTERNATIONAL INFORMATION CENTRE, Parliament Mansions, Orchard Street, S.W.1.
   President : Mrs. Margaret Sanger.
   Hon. Director : Mrs. Edith How-Martyn, M.Sc.

INDEX

Printed in Dunstable, United Kingdom

91343238R00123